Mehdi RABHIA
Hind ARZOUR
Rim KHELIFA

CMV infections in kidney transplant patients

Mehdi RABHIA
Hind ARZOUR
Rim KHELIFA

CMV infections in kidney transplant patients

ScienciaScripts

Imprint

Cover image: www.ingimage.com

This book is a translation from the original published under ISBN 978-620-6-71113-1.

Publisher:
Sciencia Scripts
is a trademark of
Dodo Books Indian Ocean Ltd. and OmniScriptum S.R.L publishing group

120 High Road, East Finchley, London, N2 9ED, United Kingdom
Str. Armeneasca 28/1, office 1, Chisinau MD-2012, Republic of Moldova, Europe
Printed at: see last page
ISBN: 978-620-8-13948-3

CONTENTS

List of abbreviations 2

Introduction 5

Literature review 7

1. Cytomegalovirus 8

2. Transplantation 20

3. CMV in kidney transplant patients 27

Conclusion 37

References 38

List of abbreviations

CMV	Cytomegalovirus
CMVH	Human cytomegalovirus
DNA	Deoxyribonucleic acid
RNA	Ribonucleic acid
Kpb	kilo Basic pairs
US	Single Short Segment
UL	Segment Long Unique
TRL	Terminal Long Repeat
IRS	Short Internal Repeat
TRS	Terminal Repeat Short
IRL	Long Internal repeat
MCP	Major Capsid Protein
MCP	Minor Capsid Protein
MCBP	Minor Capsid Binding Protein
SCP	Smallest Capsid Protein
TLR	Toll-Like Receptor
AP	Assembly protein
PP	Phosphoprotein
g (B,L,O,H,M,N)	glycoprotein (B,L,O,H,M,N)
IE	Immediate Early
RE	Endoplasmic reticulum
IL	Interleukin
SI	Immune System
NK	Natural Killer
LT	T lymphocyte
LB	B lymphocyte
CTL	Cytotoxic T Lymphocyte
CPA	Antigen Presenting Cell
TCR	T-Cell Receptor

Epo	Erythropoietin
DFG	Glomerular filtration rate
IRA	Acute renal failure
IRC	Chronic renal failure
IRT	End-stage renal failure
EER	Extra Renal Purification
RCM	Chronic kidney disease
SRAA	Renin-Angiotensin-Aldosterone System
HTA	Hypertension
TNF alpha	Tumor Necrosis Factors
CD3	Differentiation cluster 3
PCR	Polymerase Chain Reaction
CSF	Cerebrospinal fluid
GCV	Ganciclovir
VGCV	Valganciclovir
NFS	Blood cell count
HLA	Human Leukocyte Antigens
SNSF	Blood cell count
SPSS	Statistical Package for the Social Sciences
H	Men
F	Woman
THYMOG	Thymoglobulin
CICLO	Ciclosporin
TACRO	Tacrolimus
MMF	Mycophenolate Mofetil

Introduction

Renal transplantation is currently considered to be one of the best treatments for chronic renal failure, in terms of both survival and cost **(Halloran, 2004)**.

Developments and tremendous progress in the field of immunosuppression have led to a spectacular improvement in graft survival, but any immunosuppressive treatment subjects the recipient to an increased risk of infection and neoplasia **(Mourad et al., 2005).**

Infection with human cytomegalovirus (HCMV) is the most frequent infection after organ transplantation **(Cannon et al., 2010)**, and the morbidity associated with this pathology continues to pose problems despite therapeutic advances **(Weclawiak et al., 2010).**

In kidney transplantation, this viral infection remains a major problem, both in terms of its frequency and its impact on patient and graft outcome.

With this in mind, the aim of the present work is to determine the frequency of cytomegalovirus infection as a function of epidemiological characteristics, and to investigate the relationship between the onset of CMV infection and the overexpression of immunosuppression and rejection.

To this end, the first part of our work consists of a bibliographical review of general information on cytomegalovirus and its use in kidney transplantation.

The second part of this work focuses on the retrospective study on the frequency of CMV infections in kidney transplant recipients in the Nephrology Department of the Mustapha Bacha University Hospital Center over the period 2015-2018. The results are obtained following a statistical analysis of the collected data.

Literature review

1. Cytomegalovirus

1.1. History

The first description of cytomegalovirus pathogenesis dates back to the early 20th century. In 1904, Ribbert, Jesionek and Kiolemenoglou first described the presence of large cells with intranuclear inclusion in the kidneys, lungs, liver and parotid glands of fetuses and stillborn babies **(Jesionek & Kiolemenoglou, 1904)**.

In the 1920s, **Cole and Kuttner** considered the viral origin of this condition, then known as "cytomegalic inclusion disease", by showing a similarity between these lesions and the cells of varicella skin lesions, as well as the histological study of salivary glands from infected guinea pigs.

In the 1950s, the disease began to be diagnosed. Wyatt suggested the first diagnostic technique, which involved testing the urine of newborns for cells characteristic of CMV infection. In 1956, **Smith** obtained replication of the virus responsible for "cytomegalic inclusion disease" in human fibroblast cells cultured in vitro. In 1959, cmv retinitis was described for the first time. It occurred in cancer patients treated with chemotherapy and organ transplant recipients receiving immunosuppressive therapy.

In 1960, Weller et al. coined the term "cytomegalovirus" because of the morphology of the infected cells **(Weller, 1970)**. CMV was isolated for the first time from a kidney transplant patient in 1965 **(Klemola & Kaarianinen, 1965).**

Subsequent serological studies have demonstrated that cytomegalovirus infection is widespread in the global population, and that there is a link between lowered immune defenses and reactivation of the virus **(Simon, 2014).**

1.2. Classification

Herpesviruses are widely distributed viruses in the biosphere, infecting a huge number of different animal species. They all belong to the order Herpesvirales and to the three families Herpesviridae, Alloherpesviridae, and Malacoherpesviridae **(Davison et al., 2009; Agut, 2011).**

In the Herpesviridae family, 8 human-infecting viruses have been counted, classified into 3 subfamilies (alpha-, beta- and gamma *herpesvirinae)* according to their genome structure and sequence homologies. CMV is a *Betaherpesvirinae.*

According to the classification of the International Committee on Taxonomy of Viruses, updated in 2013, human cytomegalovirus or human herpesvirus 5 (CMV) belongs to the cytomegalovirus genus and is a member of the Herpesviridae family, a family characterized by its ability to infect cells latently, with periodic reactivations (**Tab.1.1**) (**Mocarski, 2001**).

Table.1.1 Classification of human herpes viruses (Crough & Khanna, 2009).

Herpesvirus	Abbreviation		Size (kb)
	Common	Formal	
Alphaherpesvirinae			
Simplexvirus			
Herpes simplex virus type 1	HSV-1	HHV-1	152
Herpes simplex virus type 2	HSV-2	HHV-2	155
Varicellovirus			
Varicella-zoster virus	VZV	HHV-3	125
Betaherpesvirinae			
Cytomegalovirus			
HCMV	HCMV	HHV-5	227–236
Roseolovirus			
Human herpesvirus type 6	HHV-6	HHV-6	159–162
Human herpesvirus type 7	HHV-7	HHV-7	144–153
Gammaherpesvirinae			
Lymphocryptovirus			
EBV	EBV	HHV-4	172–173
Rhadinovirus			
Human herpesvirus type 8	HHV-8	HHV-8	134–138

1.3. Structure of cytomegalovirus

CMV shares the same structure as all Herpesviruses, but is larger, between 200 and 300 nanometers in diameter.

The virion is mainly composed of a 235 Kbp DNA double helix protected by an icosahedral nucleocapsid, itself surrounded by the integument. The whole is covered by an envelope of cellular origin carrying numerous viral glycoproteins **(Fig.1.1) (Lammers et al., 1996; Wright et al., 1998; Brown et al., 1999).**

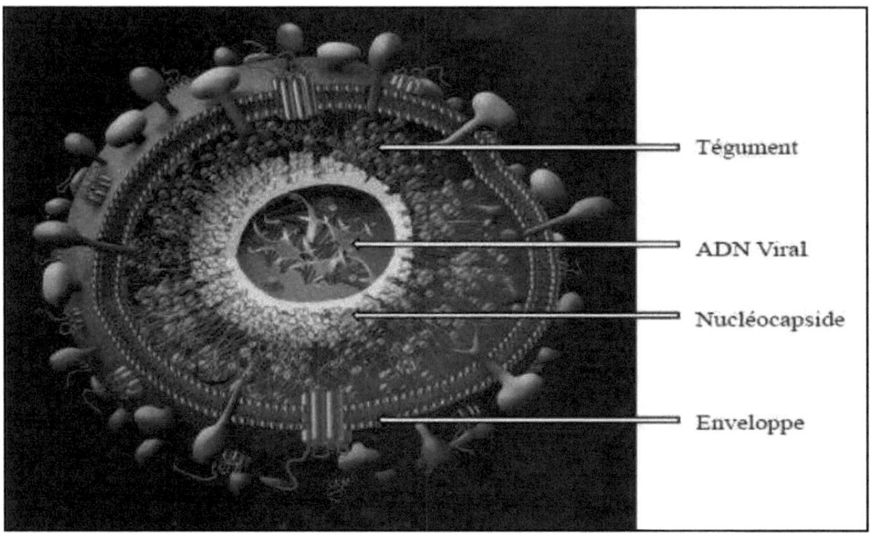

Figure 1.1 Structure of the HCMV virion (Streblow et al., 2006).

1.3.1 The genome

The viral genome is a double-stranded DNA of around 235 Kbp, the largest of all herpesviruses and one of the longest of all known human viruses **(Cha et al., 1996).** It consists of two unique segments: a unique short segment (US) and a unique long segment (UL).

The UL region accounts for 82% of the viral genome, and contains genes that play a key role in viral replication **(Sijmons et al., 2014).**

Each of these segments is flanked at its ends by terminal inverted repeats, TRLs for UL and TRSs for US. At the intersection of these two segments are two internal sequences, IRL and IRS **(Fig.1.2).**

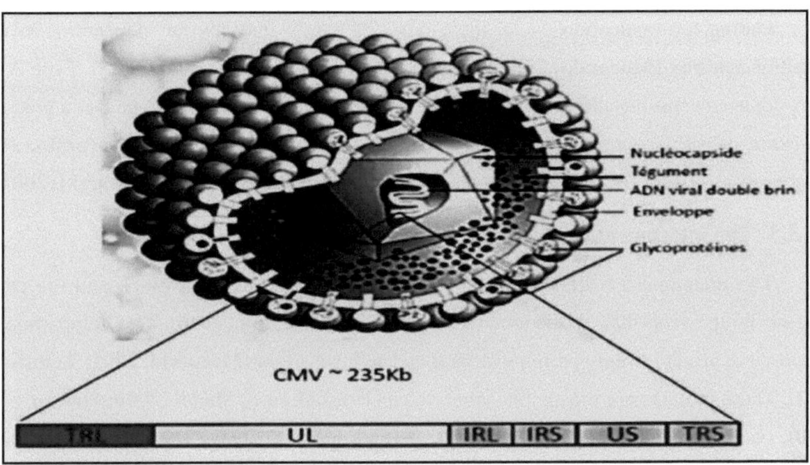

Figure.1.2 The different segments of the viral genome. TRL: Terminal Repeat Long; UL: Unique Long; IRL: Internal Repeat Long; IRS: Internal Repeat Short; US: Unique Short; TRS: Terminal Repeat Short **(Tomtishen, 2012; Crough & Khanna, 2009).**

1.3.2 The nucleocapsid

The CMV capsid is about 100 nm in diameter and comprises 162 capsomeres (subunits) arranged in icosahedral symmetry. It is made up of 7 proteins:

- The UL86 protein, known as MCP (Major Capsid Protein), is the main component of the pentamers and hexamers that form the basis of the icosahedral capsid structure. This polypeptide is one of the most conserved herpesvirus proteins.
- The UL85 protein, known as MCP (Minor Capsid Protein), is located inside the capsid and enables viral DNA to bind to it.
- The Minor Capsid Binding Protein (MCBP), encoded by the UL46 gene. It is mainly present in triplex form, and ensures the maintenance of pentamers and hexamers.
- SCP (Smallest Capsid Protein), also known as UL48/49 protein. It contributes to capsid cohesion by lining the ends of hexamers.
- Three proteins are derived from the peptide encoded by the UL80 gene. After three post-translational cleavages, the UL80 protein gives rise to proteins with distinct but complementary functions within the capsid **(Cotin, 2011).**

During the replication cycle, three types of capsid may appear, depending on their degree of maturity **(Mocarski, 2001; Gibson, 1996; Irmiere & Gibson, 1983)**. Type A is a DNA-depleted capsid resulting from a defect in viral genome packaging. Type B is a precursor of mature capsids, containing no viral DNA but the assembly proteins **(Mocarski, 2001; Butcher et al., 1998)**. Type C corresponds to fully mature nucleocapsids **(Mocarski, 2001).**

1.3.3 The integument

The integument is defined as the space between the lipid envelope and the capsid proteins. It represents 40% of the total mass of the virion **(Maude, 2016).** This compartment is composed of around twenty proteins of viral and cellular origin **(Mocarski, 2001; Tomtishen, 2012)**. These proteins are mostly phosphorylated **(Bresnahan & Shenk, 2000; Greijer et al., 2000)**, two of which are highly immunogenic and appear to play a key role in viral gene regulation and the control of cellular metabolism during viral replication. These are the pp150 (UL32) and pp65 (UL83) proteins.

The UL83 protein is found in the nucleus immediately after viral infection and associates with the nuclear matrix during the late stages of replication. It alone accounts for 15% of all integument proteins **(Simon, 2014).** It is followed by pp71, encoded by the UL82 gene and which plays an important role in replication **(Tomtishen, 2012; Liu & Stinski, 1992).**

The UL97 protein kinase appears to play a central role in CMVH infection, acting at various levels, notably in the exit of the capsid from the nucleus and the phosphorylation required for ganciclovir activation thus becoming the first target of resistance mutations to this molecule **(Simon, 2014).**

1.3.4 The viral envelope

The envelope is derived from the host cell's intracellular (nuclear and cytoplasmic) membranes: it is a lipid bilayer into which various viral glycoproteins are inserted in the form of glycoprotein complexes **(Britt & Boppana, 2004).** It has a large number of glycoproteins on its surface, the most important of which are gB, gH, gL, gO, gM and gN. The envelope confers virion sensitivity to lipid solvents, low pH and heat **(Muriel, 2010).**

The gB protein, encoded by UL55, is a transmembrane glycoprotein essential for the interaction of heparan-sulfate residues during virus entry and adhesion **(Compton et al., 1993; Britt & Mach, 1996).** It is particularly immunogenic and is the major target of neutralizing antibodies, the use of which can inhibit virus/cell attachment and fusion **(Gicklhorn et al., 2003).** It is highly conserved in CMVs of different species **(Compton et al., 1993).**

The gH protein ensures fusion of the viral envelope with the cell membrane. It is a target for neutralizing antibodies, which block membrane fusion and viral penetration **(Simpson et al., 1993).**

The gM/gN complex also allows initial interaction with heparan sulfates. The gM protein is the most abundant surface protein, accounting for 10% of virion mass. Its structure is globally conserved in Herpesviridae **(Lehner et al., 1989)**. The gN protein is highly variable from one CMV strain to another. These proteins are not essential for viral replication in vitro.

1.4. Cytomegalovirus replication

CMVH replicates only in human cells **(Descamps, 2014).** This mechanism requires interaction between a viral envelope protein and heparan sulfates on the cell surface. The viral protein that interacts most with these surface molecules is the gB protein. This virus has various glycoproteins that have been described as mediators of cell entry, and these differ according to cell type. For fibroblasts, this is the gH/gL/gO complex, while entry into epithelial and endothelial cells and monomacrophages is mediated by the gH/gL/UL128-131 pentamer **(Vanarsdall &** Johnson, 2012; Vanarsdall et al., 2016; Sathiyamoorthy et al., 2017; Gerna et al., 2017; Cui et al., 2017; Wu et al., 2017).

Entry of the viral particle occurs via binding between glycoprotein complexes of the virus and cellular receptors **(Harwardt et al., 2016).** Several of these have been identified: the Endothelial Growth Factor receptor, integrins, Platelet Derived Growth Factor, and Neuropilin-2 **(Chan et al., 2009; Feire et al., 2010; Wang et al., 2005; Soroceanu et al., 2008; Martinez-Martin et al., 2018)**, followed by fusion of the viral envelope with the cell membrane to release the nucleocapsid into the cytoplasm **(Harwardt et al., 2016).** The nucleocapsid is then translocated to the nucleus, where viral DNA is released **(Fig.1.3) (Sanchez et al., 2002).**

We then distinguish 3 different event phases:

- A **very early** phase during which the so-called Immediate Early genes are transcribed. Their regulatory proteins divert the cell's energy and resources to viral replication, and the next phase.

- An **early** phase during which most of the viral genome is available for transcription. This phase involves at least 23 early genes, which play a crucial role during replication, notably in DNA synthesis. Synthesis then begins **(Yu et al., 2005).**

- a so-called **late** phase, during which the later, mainly structural proteins are synthesized (envelope glycoproteins and capsid structural proteins). DNA is encapsulated to form the capsid in the nucleus, followed by envelopment by vesicles derived from the Golgi apparatus. Fusion of these vesicles with the cell membrane results in the exit of enveloped virions (exocytosis) **(Vanarsdall & Johnson, 2012; Paulus & Nevels, 2009; Crough & khanna, 2009).**

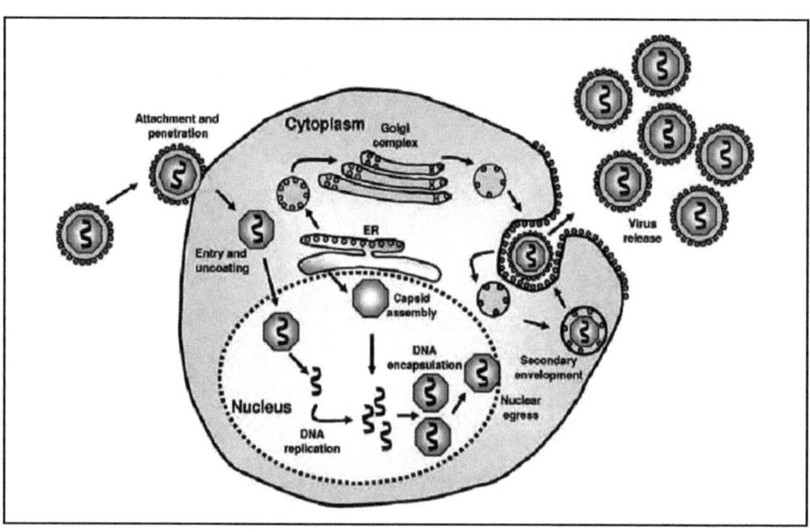

Figure 1.3 CMV lytic viral cycle. Once the nucleocapsid has been released into the cytoplasm, it is transported to the nucleus, where viral DNA is replicated following prior expression of the IE1 and IE2 genes. In the later phases of the cycle, viral DNA is encapsidated before being enveloped once by the nuclear membrane and then a second time by the ER membrane. Virions are then released by exocytosis **(Crough & Khanna, 2009).**

1.5. Transmission mode

Humans are the only reservoir of the virus (**Kurath & Resch, 2010**), and transmission is exclusively human-to-human, requiring direct mucosal contact with infectious bodily fluids such as urine, saliva and semen (**Kapranos et al., 2003**), as well as vaginal secretions (**Ludwig & Hengel, 2009**).

CMV is the only herpes virus that can be transmitted from mother to fetus or newborn. This is the most widespread form of transmission, maintaining the virus population worldwide **(Reynolds et al., 1973).**

Blood products and transplanted organs are the main vectors of CMV transmission in hospitals. Transmission by blood donation is also possible **(Lowance et al., 1999).**

1.6. Pathophysiology

CMVH is a lytic virus with a cytopathic effect that actively replicates and disseminates its viremia throughout the body's various organs, i.e. its viral genome remains indefinitely in target cells.

Depending on host immunity, it can reactivate, multiply and cause severe multi-visceral damage. When the host's immune system is strong, the primary infection is usually asymptomatic. Occasionally, symptoms such as fever, cervical adenopathy, pharyngitis and fatigue appear (**Esclatine & Géniteau, 2002**).

1.6.1 Cellular tropism and blood dissemination

In vivo, the cellular tropism of CMVH is highly varied. It can be acquired via the hematogenous route (transplantation or transfusion of blood products), or enter mucous membranes and spread in the transitory bloodstream, enabling the virus to reach its target organs.

This ability to disseminate throughout the body is linked to the multiplicity of cell types that the virus can infect (endothelial, epithelial and fibroblastic cells). Once these target cells have been reached, the virus spreads from cell to cell **(Anne-Laure, 2013).**

CMVH replicates in fibroblastic cells, endothelial cells, epithelial cells, muscle cells, nerve cells and macrophages, enabling it to infect a wide range of tissues and organs **(Sinzger et al., 1995).** This broad tropism explains the diversity of clinical signs encountered.

The virus is disseminated mainly via infection of endothelial cells, monocytes, macrophages and polynuclear cells.

Tissue dissemination from viremia occurs via several mechanisms:

- The secretion of cytokines such as interleukin-8 (IL-8) by endothelial cells enables polynuclear recruitment **(Gretchen et al., 2008).**
- Through direct cell-to-cell contact, these polynuclei acquire mature virions and the nuclear-targeted pUL83 (pp65) protein.
- Infected endothelial cells transmit the virus to circulating monocytes, which in turn transmit the virus to uninfected cells.

- Monocytes become capable of replicating the virus when they differentiate into macrophages, which can disseminate the virus into tissues.
- Infected endothelial cells can themselves induce organ infection when they detach, circulate and are sequestered due to their size in capillaries **(Anne-Laure, 2013).**

1.6.2 Latency and reactivation of CMVH

After primary infection, HCMV persists within the host. Many organs harbor the virus in a latent state. Nevertheless, latency is established preferentially in monocytes and macrophages, but also in endothelial cells **(Ligat, 2017).**

Viral DNA, which remains latent as an episome in target cells, can also be reactivated at any time. This is known as secondary reactivation infection **(Willam, 2019).**

The host immune system plays an important role in the latency process and in virus reactivation. Indeed, immunosuppression can lead to reactivation of the virus, resulting in new viremia **(Sinclair & Sissons, 2006; Söderberg-Nauclér et al., 1997).**

In immunocompetent individuals, CMVH infection often goes unnoticed, but in highly immunocompromised individuals it can lead to serious illness.

In pregnant women, there is a relative immunosuppression, which plays a potential role in CMV reactivations. It is also possible to become infected with a different strain of the virus. This is known as secondary reinfection **(Cannon & Davis, 2005).**

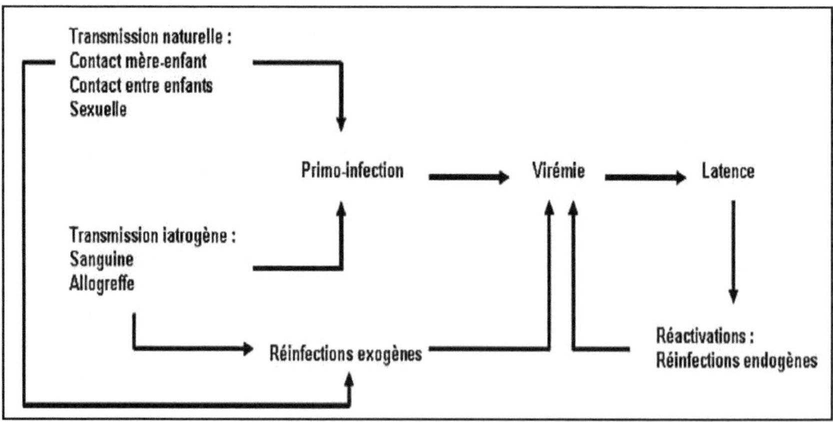

Figure.1.4 Pathophysiology of CMV infection (**Alain & Mazeron, 2003**).

1.7. Anti-CMV immunity

CMV infection leads to the activation of an immune response that confers protection against the virus (**Lucie, 2013**). As both innate and adaptive (humoral and cellular) responses are involved in the process, they work together to fight HCMV effectively. On the other hand, the immune system is unable to prevent the early stages of viral infection and the establishment of latency, meaning that the virus can persist throughout an individual's life.

1.7.1 Innate immunity

The innate immune response constitutes a first barrier to viral infection and plays an important role in direct defense against CMV (**Compton et al., 2003**). It kicks in as soon as the virus attaches and fuses to the cell's plasma membrane **(Boehme et al., 2006).**

Activation of the innate immune system induces the production of pro-inflammatory cytokines (**Tabeta et al., 2004; Compton et al., 2003**), leading to the activation of macrophages, Natural Killer (NK) cells and dendritic cells.

- NK activity increases during the acute phase of infection, but also during reactivations, indicating the contribution of NKs to HCMV infection (**Venema et al., 1949**). By releasing perforins and granzyme, they lyse infected cells **(Vivier et al., 2008).**
- Dendritic cells are among the first cells infected at the various sites of viral entry during primary infection **(Crough & Khanna, 2009).**

1.7.2 Adaptive immunity

The players in adaptive immunity are LTs and LBs. The two essential features of the adaptive immune system are an extremely diverse antigen recognition repertoire (several million specificities) and the ability to establish a memory response.

This general feature of the adaptive immune response confers on the immune system its ability to rapidly prevent or control secondary infections by genetically closely related viruses **(Boppana et al., 2001).** However, CMV is a notable exception to this rule. Indeed, it can repeatedly establish persistent infections in immunocompetent hosts. This ability is probably the reason for the presence of different HCMV genotypes in the same individual **(Meyer-Konig et al., 1998).**

1.7.2.1 Cell-mediated immunity

In response to infection, T-cell-mediated immunity acts predominantly against CMVH viral replication. Although the virus is not eradicated by the immune response, CD4+, CD8+ T cells play an important role in controlling and limiting CMV replication.

1.7.2.1.1 T-CD4 lymphocytes

Numerous studies show the major role played by CD4+ lymphocytes in the fight against CMV **(Tu et al., 2004).**

LT CD4+ or helper lymphocytes play a central, even indispensable role in adaptive immunity, activating the humoral response by cooperating with LBs to induce their differentiation into plasma cells, as well as the cytotoxic response via LT CD8+ that differentiate into CTL (cytotoxic T lymphocyte).

Following CMVH infection, LT helper cells recognize CMV-specific epitopes on the surface of antigen-presenting cells (APCs) (macrophages, dendritic cells or B lymphocytes) via their T-Cell Receptor (TCR). Internalization of the TCR/antigen complex, under the action of interleukin 1 produced by APCs, leads to the production of CD4+helper LT clones specific to the detected CMV epitope.

These LTs will activate the cytotoxic T response via their production of cytokines such asinterleukin 2, 12or IFN-γ, and activate B lymphocytes via their secretion of interleukins IL-4, 5, 10 and 13 **(Lucie, 2013).**

In 2002, **Einsele et al** showed that CD4+ cells are necessary for the control of CMV infection. In their study, the transfer of CMV-specific CD4+ cell lines drastically reduced viral load in stem cell transplant p a t i e n t s , and also contributed to the expansion of CD8+ cells.

1.7.2.1.2 T-CD8 lymphocytes

CD8 + lymphocyte activity is dependent on cytokines such as IFN-γ and IL- 2, produced by CD4 + TL (**Gamadia et al., 2003**). Following this stimulation, CD8 + LT produce cytotoxic mediators such as perforin and granzyme B, which cause membrane damage to the host cell.

Memory CD8+ T lymphocytes, sensitized to CMV proteins, persist in the body.

1.7.2.2 Humoral-mediated immunity

Primary CMV infection leads to the synthesis of antibodies directed against various viral proteins. In particular, these antibodies are directed against integument proteins (pp65, pp150), envelope proteins (gB, gH, gM/gN) or non-structural proteins such as IE1.

Most antibodies observed in CMV-positive individuals are directed against envelope glycoproteins, and over 50% of these are neutralizing antibodies that recognize a gB epitope (**Macagno et al., 2010**). The importance of CMV-specific humoral immunity remains poorly understood, but it appears to restrict viral dissemination and limit the severity of clinical manifestations.

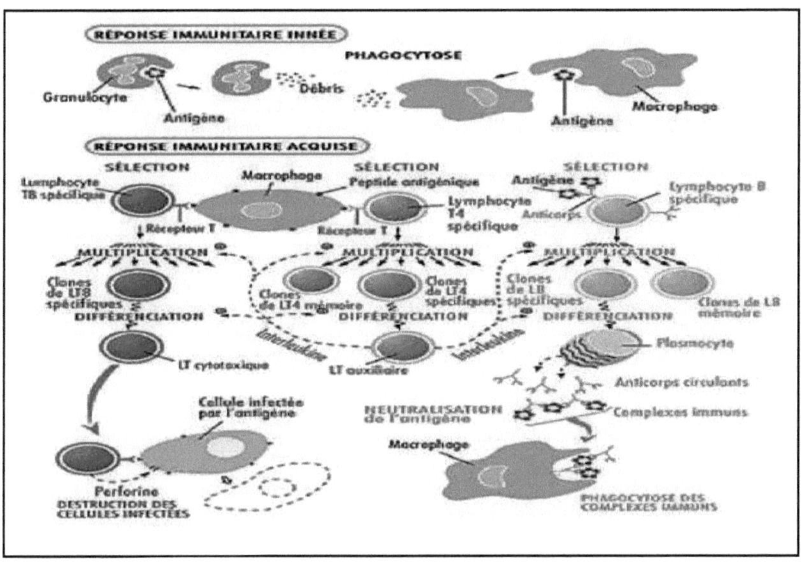

Figure.1.5 Innate and acquired immune responses **(Lucie, 2013).**

2. Transplantation

2.1. Anatomical and historical overview of the kidney

The kidneys are two bean-shaped organs, each weighing around 100 to 200 grams **(Johann et al., 2013).**

Each kidney is covered by a relatively strong, smooth, fibrous renal capsule, which contains the renal parenchyma in two parts: a peripheral part, the cortex, and a central part, the medulla.

In the medulla, we find a set of pyramidal structures called Malpighi pyramids, whose base touches the surface of the kidney and is thus covered by the cortex, and whose apex constitutes the renal papillae found in the medulla (**Lacour, 2013**).

Renal pyramids numbering 8 to 12 per kidney are separated by cortical tissue this separation forms renal columns called bertin columns, a pyramid with the two surrounding columns forms a renal lobe **(Johann et al., 2013).**

The renal cortex extends from the renal capsule to the base of the pyramids, but also between them.

The renal parenchyma contains around 1 to 1.5 million nephrons per kidney; these are the kidney's functional units, and will be responsible for urine production **(Lacour, 2013).**

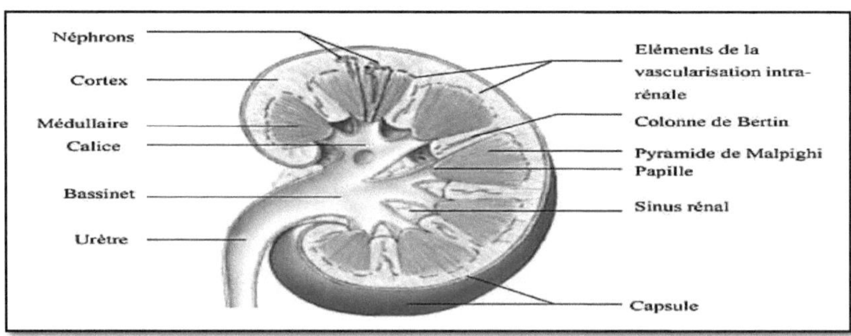

Figure.2.6 Anatomy of a kidney **(Bernard, 2013).**

2.2. Reminder of physiology

The kidneys are the organs where the main functions of the urinary system are performed, as the other parts of the system are primarily conduíts and storage sites (**Tortora & Grabowski, 2001**). They perform both endocrine and exocrine functions.

2.2.1 Function endocrine

The kidney acts as an endocrine gland, secreting substances such as..:

- The factor erythropoietin (Epo) in their secretion stimulates the production of red blood cells by the bone marrow.
- Renin, an enzyme that activates the renin-angiotensin-aldosterone system, is involved in regulating blood pressure.
- Prostaglandin increases glomerular blood flow and glomerular filtration rate. **(Tortora & Grabowski, 2001).**

The kidney is also the site of transformation of vitamin D into its active metabolites **(Guyton Arthur, 1998).**

2.2.2 Function exocrine

Exocrine function: urine production, elimination of waste products and maintenance of ionic balance.

2.2.2.1 Urine formation

Formed in nephrons by a complex three-stage process: glomerular filtration, tubular resorption, tubular secretion **(Bernard, 2013).**

2.2.2.1.1 Glomerular filtration

Glomerular filtration is the first stage in urine production. It takes place in the renal corpuscles through the glomerular membrane under hydrostatic pressure (**Tortora & Angnostakos, 1988**). This complex structure is permeable to water and small organic molecules, but retains cells and most macromolecules such as proteins, fatty acids, many drugs and a fraction of plasma calcium **(Querin & Valiquite, 2000)**. Selection is based on both molecule size and ionic charge.

The filtra obtained ends up in the glomerular chamber has a composition identical to that of blood plasma (same concentration for each element as in plasma), it's called primitive urine **(Dennai, 2012).**

Total filtration therefore depends on the number of nephrons and the glomerular filtration rate (GFR), estimated at 120 mL/min/1.73 m2 in a healthy young adult **(Daroux et al, 2009).**

2.2.2.1.2 Tubular reabsorption and secretion

Reabsorption consists in the passage of substances useful to the body that must not be eliminated, such as water, from the tubular lumen into the interstitial space and then into the peri-tubular capillaries.

Secretion is the opposite of reabsorption. The main substances eliminated by this phenomenon (urea, uric acid and potassium) move from the capillaries, interstitial space or tubular cells into the tubular lumen (**Mombazet, 2010**).

Through the formation of urine, the kidneys help excrete waste products, i.e. substances that have no useful function in the body.

Other kidney functions:

- γ Regulation of blood concentrations of several ions (Na^+ , K^+ , Ca^{++} , Cl^-) **(Tortora & Grabowski, 2001).**
- γ Maintains the body's water balance.
- γ Maintenance of appropriate osmolarity of body fluids primarily by adjusting water elimination **(Sherwood, 2006).**
- γ Regulation of intra- and extracellular blood volume and acid-base status **(Gueutin, 2012).**

2.3. Renal insufficiency

2.3.1 Definition

Renal failure is defined as a pathological state in which the kidneys function below normal levels in relation to their ability to evacuate waste, concentrate urine and maintain hydro-electrolyte balance, blood pressure and calcium metabolism **(Dussol, 2011).**

Renal function can **deteriorate rapidly** (known as **acute renal failure [ARF]**) or **progressively** (known as **chronic renal failure [CRF]**). Sometimes it can even lead to **end-stage renal disease (ESRD), which requires supplementary treatment** (extra-renal cleansing (EER)) by hemodialysis or peritoneal dialysis and/or kidney transplantation.

Chronic kidney disease (CKD) is defined by the progressive and irreversible decline in glomerular filtration rate (GFR), which is the best indicator of renal function. It usually results from the evolution of chronic kidney disease (CKD) **(Moulin & Peraldi, 2016).**

It is defined as a glomerular filtration rate < 60 ml/min/1.73m² of body surface area for more than three months. Renal function is measured by an endogenous marker, creatinine, which is a degradation product of skeletal muscle creatine, essentially eliminated renally via glomerular filtration and to a lesser extent via tubular secretion. Renal function can be estimated either by creatinine clearance or by calculating glomerular filtration rate **(Bordage, 2015).**

2.3.2 Consequences of end-stage renal disease

In **CKD,** the kidney no longer performs its main functions of excreting waste products from nitrogen metabolism, regulating the electrolyte balance and producing hormones.

2.3.2.1 Uremic syndrome

The elimination of urea and other nitrogen products formed by protein catabolism is mainly renal.

The concentration of urea in the blood is proportional to the degree of renal failure, defined as a reduction in the number of functional nephrons. When urea levels exceed 40mmol/l (the norm is 2.8-7.6mmol/l), uremic syndrome develops, causing nausea, vomiting, asthenia and impaired concentration, anorexia and cramping **(Man et al, 2010).**

2.3.2.2 Loss of hydroelectrolytic functions

Regulation of the body's water and electrolyte balance is preserved until the end stage of renal failure, thanks to hyperfiltration. When only 5% of nephrons are functional, this adaptation is no longer possible. At this stage, dialysis is essential to the patient's survival.

2.3.2.3 Loss of endocrine functions

CKD results in reduced production of erythropoietin and 1-alpha-hydroxylase. This decrease is responsible for anemia and phosphocalcic disorders requiring specific pharmacological treatment. On the other hand, the renin-angiotensin-aldosterone system (RAAS) is generally exacerbated in these patients, contributing to hypertension **(Man et al, 2010).**

2.4. Treatments

Once the stage of chronic end-stage renal failure has been reached, suppletive treatment must be rapidly considered and implemented to eliminate the waste products that will accumulate in the body, and to ensure the body's homeostasis by maintaining hydroelectrolytic and acid-base balance (the kidney's endocrine and exocrine functions) **(Petitclerc, 1998; Canaud et al, 2005; Vincent & Pierre, 2006).**

There are two types of replacement technology:

- Dialysis;
- Kidney transplantation.

2.4.1 Dialysis

The elimination of a certain number of molecules (ions, products of nitrogen catabolism, drugs) as well as water is ensured by extrarenal purification. There are two types, each requiring a specific approach:

- Vascular: arteriovenous fistula for hemodialysis;
- Peritoneal: peritoneal dialysis catheter for peritoneal dialysis.

2.4.2 Transplantation

Of all the treatments for chronic kidney disease, renal transplantation is indisputably the one that brings patients not only a better quality of life, but also prolonged survival **(Sayegh & Carpenter, 2004).** It can be considered for any patient with chronic renal failure, whether already on dialysis or with dialysis imminent (pre-emptive transplant), provided that the patient expresses the will to undergo transplantation, that the risks involved do not exceed the expected benefits, and that there are no contraindications **(Knoll, 2013).**

The pre-transplant protocol at Mustapha Bacha Hospital is as follows: clinical, biological and morphological assessment.

2.4.2.1 Complications of kidney transplantation

2.4.2.1.1 Delayed return to work (RRF)

In most cases, the graft resumes diuresis immediately or in the hours following surgery, with improvement in renal function.

However, in around 20-30% of cases, this recovery of function is delayed (from a few days to 3 or 4 weeks), with the formation of an ARF. In less than 5% of cases, the RRF is irreversible: this is known as "primary graft non-function" or "non-viable graft" (**Mourad et al., 2005**).

The need for dialysis in the first week after transplantation seems to be the most commonly accepted criterion until diuresis and then function return.

2.4.2.1.2 Risk of rejection

Rejection corresponds to the induction of an immune response by the recipient against the transplanted organ. Rejection leads to more or less rapid destruction of the transplanted organ in the absence of immunosuppressive treatment. There are three types of rejection: hyperacute rejection, acute rejection which may be humoral or cellular, and chronic rejection. These raise highly complex and sometimes interrelated diagnostic and therapeutic issues **(Anglicheau et al., 2007).**

2.4.2.1.2.1 Hyperacute rejection

Hyperacute rejection generally occurs within the first 24 hours after transplantation. It is essentially linked to the presence, in the serum of the "immune" recipient, of lymphocytotoxic anti-HLA antibodies produced in response to blood transfusions, pregnancies or previous transplants **(Anglicheau et al., 2007).**

2.4.2.1.2.2 Acute rejection

Acute cellular rejection, which generally occurs in the first few months after transplantation. It is the most frequently observed type of rejection, accounting for around 80% of acute rejection episodes. CD4+ and CD8+ T cells are incriminated in its occurrence **(Kaboré, 2017).**

Humoral acute rejection occurs mainly between the first and third week post-transplant, but can also occur later. This type of rejection is due to the appearance of antibodies specifically directed against antigenic determinants of the donor. The diagnosis should be made in the presence o f either delayed recovery of renal function or early acute renal failure **(Anglicheau et al., 2007; Legendre et al., 2010).**

2.4.2.1.2.3 Chronic rejection

Now known as chronic graft nephropathy, it is the main cause of renal graft loss, particularly in the long term. Chronic graft rejection is caused by two main groups of factors. Immunological factors, which are identical to those incriminated in the occurrence of hyper-acute and acute rejection, and non-immunological factors (donor-inherited lesions, nephrotoxicity of immunosuppressants, post-ischemic lesions, infections, hypertension, diabetes, recurrence of initial graft disease **(Anglicheau et al., 2007).**

The considerable progress made over the last 20 years is due to the combined effect of a very significant reduction in the incidence of acute rejection, a testament to the effectiveness of immunosuppression **(Hariharan et al., 2003; Alonso & Oliver, 2004).**

The principle of immunosuppression in renal transplantation is to prevent acute rejection. This is based on:

- induction therapy, which consists in combining immunosuppressive treatments with polyclonal anti-lymphocytic antibodies or an interleukin-2 receptor antagonist.
- maintenance treatment, which is more intense during the first three months after transplantation. It is gradually modified thereafter to reduce the risk of adverse effects and improve tolerance of long-term immunosuppressive therapy without risking graft rejection **(Balsa et al., 2011; Abramovicz et al., 2000).**

2.4.2.1.3 Risk of infection

Renal transplant patients are at high risk of infection due to three factors: immunosuppression, the nature and number of invasive procedures they undergo, and exposure to community-acquired or nosocomial germs **(Mamzer-Brunee, 2008).**

During the first month, the risk of infection is dominated by nosocomial infections, infections originating from the donor, or latent infections in the recipient. Between the second and sixth months, reactivations of latent infections and the first opportunistic infections may appear. From the sixth month onwards, the level of therapeutic immunosuppression is less intense, prophylactic treatments are generally discontinued, and kidney transplant patients are mainly exposed to infectious risks from community-acquired germs. Nevertheless, the risk of opportunistic infection remains real. These infections may be fungal, bacterial or viral, such as **cytomegalovirus infections (Anglicheau et al., 2007; Mamzer-Brunee, 2008).**

3. CMV in kidney transplant patients

3.1. Epidemiology

CMV infection is endemic, occurring throughout the year with no seasonal upsurge. Primary infection generally occurs in infancy, through contact with body fluids such as blood, saliva, tears and breast milk **(Imbert, 2002).**

Seroprevalence varies worldwide according to factors such as age, parity, gender (in some studies, women have a higher prevalence), geographical location, ethnic origin and socio-economic factors, with prevalence inversely correlated: developed countries have seroprevalence rates of around less than 20% in children , **(Segondy, 2009)** ranging from 40 to 60% of the adult population and 80% in the elderly population while countries in Africa and Asia, South East can reach 100% seroprevalence **(Julie, 2015).**

In organ transplantation, CMV infection is a frequent and serious opportunistic pathology, responsible for significant morbidity and mortality. The risk of infection varies according to the type of organ transplanted. The incidence of CMV infection in kidney transplant recipients is estimated at between 8 and 32% **(Patel & Paya, 1997),** rising to almost 70% at 3 months post-transplant in the absence of prophylaxis in high-risk groups (D+/R- or D+/R+) **(Sagedel et al., 2000).**

3.2. Presentation clinical

The clinical manifestations of CMV infections are polymorphous and depend largely on the level of immunosuppression. In organ transplantation, two effects are classically distinguished: direct (CMV disease) and less well-proven indirect (rejection, infections by other microorganisms, graft dysfunction) **(Anne & Victoria, 2019).**

3.2.1 Effects

CMV disease in transplant patients may be due either to acquisition from the transplanted organ or to reactivation of a latent virus in the recipient **(Doublie et al., 1999).**

This pathology is defined as CMVH-positive viremia accompanied by clinical symptoms. The latter are manifested by a CMVH syndrome (an acute, systemic illness), initially **accompanied** by fever and malaise, and frequently associated with leukopenia and thrombocytopenia **(Paya et al., 2004).**

Symptoms in the transplanted organ are then observed, such as pneumonia, gastrointestinal lesions, hepatitis, myocarditis or retinitis **(Doublie et al., 1999).**

3.2.2 Effects indirect

In addition to its direct pathogenic effects on a target organ, CMV remains associated with morbidity linked to the "**indirect effects**" of the virus **(Kamar et al., 2007).** These effects are associated with:

- Graft rejection. Following kidney transplantation, the application of immunosuppressive therapy designed to limit the risk of graft rejection, the accumulation of the latter thus strongly favors CMV replication from infections of exogenous origin, graft contamination or reactivation of a latent strain, which can lead to various changes within immune cells favoring acute rejection **(Salvadori et al., 2005; Alain & Mazeron, 2001).**
- Chronic renal graft dysfunction is also accelerated by CMV infection **(Inkinen et al., 2005).**
- Development of insulin resistance or diabetes after transplantation (Rodriguez et al., 2000; Doublie et al., 1999).

These effects occur even when viremia is low, and are thought to be linked to an immunomodulatory action of the virus in the host **(Fishman, 2007).**

In the absence of prophylaxis, infection most often occurs between the 1st and 4th month post-transplant, when immunosuppression is at its most severe. However, thanks to the use of prophylactic treatment, infection now appears later in the first year. This is why, in at-risk patients (D+/R- or R+), monthly CMV monitoring is recommended during the 1st post-transplant year **(Humar & Michaels, 2006).**

3.3. Risk factors

The most important risk factor in kidney transplantation is the recipient's pre-transplant serological status, which determines the incidence and severity of disease.

In fact, a seronegative recipient receiving a CMV-positive organ (D+/R-) may develop a primary infection.

The same applies in the case of a CMV-negative organ transplant in a seronegative (D-/R-) recipient undergoing post-transplant contamination (independent of the transplant itself).

Furthermore, transplantation of a CMV-positive graft into a seronegative or seropositive (D+/R- or D+/R+) recipient may be associated with reactivation of an endogenous strain or infection by an exogenous strain **(Metselaar & Weinarn, 1989; Wiesner et al. 1993; Pass, 2004; Rowshani et al. 2005).**

The incidence of CMV disease in transplant patients also varies according to:

- γ Use o f anti-lymphocyte serum or anti-CD3 monoclonal antibodies

  (Mourad et al., 2004).
- γ The recipient's advanced age **(Wéclawiak et al., 2004).**
- γ Acute or chronic graft rejection **(Fietze et al., 1994; Kamar et al., 2008**).
- γ Infectious stress situations (**Cook et al., 1998**).

3.4. Diagnosis of CMV infection

Diagnosis of cytomegalovirus infection helps define and limit the risks associated with CMV infection and disease. The choice of diagnosis depends on the status of each patient. Several detection and/or quantification techniques can be used: virus detection on fibroblast culture, antigen detection by immunofluorescence, nucleic acid detection by real-time PCR or immunoglobulin detection in patient blood (serology) **(Lucie, 2013).**

The diagnostic techniques for CMV infection listed below are based on the search for clinical signs, the virus, its antigens, DNA or RNA **(Gandhi & Khanna, 2004).**

3.4.1 Diagnosis direct

3.4.1.1 Cell cultures

The traditional method for detecting HCMV is cell culture. This approach uses clinical samples inoculated onto human fibroblastic cells, incubated and observed over a period ranging from 2 to 21 days. In a standard culture technique, the presence of HCMV is characterized by the appearance of foci of cells that have lost their normal spindle-shaped appearance and become rounded: this is the cytopathic effect of HCMV **(Leruez-Ville, 2001).**

However, this method is no longer used in routine diagnostics as it is slow and requires three weeks for a result to be considered negative, but retains interest for isolating strains and studying their antiviral resistance **(Kotton et al., 2013).**

3.4.1.2 Antigenemia pp65

Antigen detection techniques, such as pp65 antigenemia, are gradually being abandoned. However, they are still of interest for detecting infection in tissues **(Kotton et al., 2013).**

This simple technique is used to detect and quantify CMV viremia (i.e. the number of circulating blood cells infected with CMVH in the replicative phase). Blood is collected in a tube containing an anticoagulant and, after lysis of the red blood cells, the leukocytes are deposited on a slide. The presence of HCMV in leukocytes is revealed by immunofluorescence using monoclonal antibodies directed against the coat protein pp65. Positive cells show characteristic nuclear fluorescence **(Leruez-Ville, 2001).**

3.4.1.3 Gene amplification (polymerase chain reaction or PCR)

Molecular biology techniques are virtually the only ones used for diagnosing CMVH infections and monitoring patients. Compared with cell culture techniques or pp65 antigenemia, they have the advantage of being fast, sensitive and automatable.

These techniques can be performed on a wide range of samples (plasma, leukocytes, urine, CSF, biopsies, amniotic fluid) **(Leruez-Ville, 2001).**

3.4.1.3.1 Qualitative PCR techniques 3.

3.4.1.3.1.1 Detection of viral DNA by PCR

These techniques are highly sensitive. Various commercial kits are currently available.

The advantage of these techniques is their excellent sensitivity. This type of test is an invaluable tool in all cases where the presence of HCV needs to be detected without the risk of false negatives. These techniques detect CMVH DNA, whether from replicating or latent viruses.

3.4.1.3.1.2 Detection of viral RNA by PCR

These techniques are based on the amplification of viral messenger RNA, and detect only viruses in the active replication phase.

3.4.1.3.2 Quantitative PCR techniques

Quantitative PCR is used to monitor response to treatment and detect clinical or viral resistance.

These techniques are based on TaqMan real-time PCR technology. They enable viral load to be measured and monitored in transplant patients: the result is expressed in copies/mL of blood or units/mL of blood, and converted to log base 10 for easy comparison between two samples. A significant increase in viral load (>0.5 log) or a high initial value is indicative of CMVH infection or viral reactivation.

3.4.2 Indirect diagnosis "Serology

Serology establishes whether or not the patient has had prior contact with CMV (encounter marker). In practice, pre-transplant serology should be performed on both the donor (D) and the recipient (R) to establish D/R status and guide preventive measures. After transplantation, serology has little clinical utility **(Humar et al., 2005; Kotton et al., 2013).**

Anti-CMVH IgM can be detected by immunocapture ELISA tests; anti-CMVH IgM is only present in around 70% of primary infections in immunocompetent subjects. Anti-CMVH IgM can persist for up to 16 to 20 weeks after primary infection; however, it should be remembered that they are not specific to primary infection, since they can also be detected during CMVH viral reactivation.

The detection of anti-CMVH IgG is currently carried out using commercial ELISA kits based on recombinant proteins or synthetic peptides **(Leruez-Ville, 2001).**

3.5. Treatment

3.5.1 Antiviral molecules

The severity of CMV infection in the immunocompromised has prompted researchers to develop antiviral molecules, including Ganciclovir, Valganciclovir and Foscarnet, which are most frequently used in kidney transplant patients. The use of these molecules prevents the virus from replicating, rather than eradicating it in its latent state. Moreover, prolonged treatment, sometimes at reduced dosage, may be necessary for as long as immunodepression persists **(Gael, 2006).**

3.5.1.1 Ganciclovir (GCV) and valganciclovir (Val-GCV)

Ganciclovir (9-(1, 3-dihydroxy 2-propoxy) methyl guanine, known under the trade name Cymevan®) is an active inhibitor of herpesviruses and is the gold standard treatment for CMV infections **(Matthews & Boehme, 1988; Kotton et al., 2013).** As GCV is only active in its triphosphorylated form, it is first phosphorylated by a virus-derived serine/threonine kinase, phosphoprotein pUL97 **(Littler et al., 1992),** then GCV monophosphate (GCV-P) is taken up by two cellular kinases, guanylate kinase and phosphoglycerate kinase to become active in the triphosphated GCV-PPP form.

The latter is then recognized by the viral polymerase pUL54 as a nitrogenous base and integrated into viral DNA **(Brestrich et al., 2009)**, acting preferentially at the catalytic site of the viral DNA polymerase pUL54, in competition with the enzyme's natural nucleoside substrates and thus inhibiting elongation of the DNA molecule under synthesis by blocking the catalytic site **(Matthews & Boehme, 1988).** Virus replication is thus inhibited.

In vitro, the concentration of ganciclovir at which viral replication is inhibited by 50% (C150) is 0.7 µg/mL **(Perrottet et al., 2009).** Over 90% of ganciclovir is found in unmetabolized form in urine **(Roche, 2014).**

Ganciclovir can be administered both intravenously and orally. Its low oral bioavailability, which does not exceed 10%, has been compensated for by the development of its prodrug, valganciclovir (val-GCV), whose oral bioavailability is around 60% **(Wang et al., 2004).**

Valganciclovir is an L-valyl ester of ganciclovir **(Kotton et al., 2013).** It is recognized as a substrate by the intestinal transporter PEPT-1 and then hydrolyzed to amino acid esters by valacyclovirase hydrolases **(Layl et al., 2008).** The molecule is metabolized to ganciclovir in the intestinal wall and liver.

Numerous adverse effects are associated with the administration of GCV or its prodrug val-GCV. Among the most frequently reported is hematological toxicity, reversible on discontinuation of treatment, manifested by severe leukoneutropenia (affecting 40% of patients after 3 months of intravenous treatment) and thrombocytopenia (15% of patients after 3 months) **(Hantz et al., 2009).**

3.5.1.2 Foscarnet or phosphonoformate (PFA)

In cases of proven resistance to ganciclovir, or i n patients unable to be treated with GCV due to neutropenia (reduced blood counts) or leukopenia (reduced total blood leukocytes), foscarnet is the recommended treatment for CMVH infection in immunocompromised patients **(Kotton et al., 2010; Humar & Snydman, 2009).**

This treatment is an analogue of inorganic pyrophosphate. It is a selective and reversible competitive inhibitor of the DNA polymerase of several herpesviruses. It attaches to the pyrophosphate-binding site of pUL54 DNA polymerase, inducing suppression of viral replication **(Crumpacker, 1992; Wagstaff & Bryson, 1994)** and thus prevents the cleavage of deoxyribonucleoside triphosphates into deoxyribonucleoside diphosphates and inorganic pyrophosphates **(Wagstaff & Bryson, 1994; Hitchcock et al., 1996; Reusser, 1996).** The nucleotide cannot then be added to the elongating viral DNA chain, and viral replication is halted **(Hantz et al., 2009).** Unlike GCV, foscarnet does not require the intervention of the UL97 protein kinase, so it is active even when this viral kinase is mutated **(Jabs et al., 1998).**

The main adverse effects of this molecule affect renal function **(Torres & Boucher, 2008).** These disturbances often lead to other disorders: hypocalcemia, anemia or seizures **(Gandhi et al., 2004),** and can thus be the cause of neurological and cardiac problems **(Biron, 2006).** Other undesirable effects, such as nausea and vomiting, genital ulcerations...

3.5.2 Therapeutic strategies

Treatment strategies for CMV disease vary according to the severity of clinical manifestations. VGCV and GCV are the two first-line agents.

3.5.2.1 Preventive treatment

Universal anti-CMV prophylaxis is an approach generally reserved for at-risk patients. Antiviral therapy is started as soon as possible after transplantation and continues for several months to prevent HCV disease. This therapy generally involves the D+/R- group to prevent primary infection, less frequently the D+/R+ group to minimize reactivation of latent virus or reinfection by other genotypes, and occasionally the D-/R+ group to prevent reactivations **(Pierre, 2012).**

The major problem with a continuous preventive strategy is the appearance of late-onset HCMV. This is defined as the onset of HCMV disease after antiviral prophylaxis has been discontinued. For 3-month preventive strategies, HCMV disease usually occurs 3 to 6 months post-transplant, or sometimes later. Late-onset HCMV disease may go undiagnosed. This is often due to patients moving away from their original transplant center. Late-onset HCMV disease contributes to increased morbidity and mortality. The incidence of late-onset HCMV disease in a standard 3-month prophylaxis program is 17% to 37% in D+/R- patients **(Paya et al, 2004).**

3.5.2.2 Pre-emptive treatment

Pre-emptive therapy is undertaken to treat subjects who develop an asymptomatic active infection detected biologically by pp65 antigenemia or PCR prior to the development of CMV disease. Treatment is then carried out by oral administration of VGCV, at a dose of 900 mg/12h, or by intravenous administration of GCV, at a dose of 5 mg/Kg/12h, or PFA at a dose of 90 mg/Kg/12h. This therapeutic choice requires close virological monitoring of transplant patients **(Cotin, 2011).**

The pre-emptive strategy has the advantage of targeting a certain group of patients, and helps reduce product costs and toxicity **(Simon, 2014).** Threshold values for initiation of preemptive therapy must be validated by the transplant center prior to the start of the preemptive protocol **(Humar et al., 1999).**

3.5.2.3 Curative treatment

Curative treatment is initiated only when clinical signs of CMV disease appear. It consists of the administration of antiviral treatments active against CMV **(Fabien, 2015).**

In patients with severe CMVH disease, treatment is based on intravenous Ganciclovir **(Anne-Laure, 2013).** This molecule gives good results in transplant patients, immunosuppressed following anti-rejection treatments **(Jacobson, 1994),** the recommended dosage by this route is 5 mg/kg/12h **(Crumpacker, 1996; Biron, 2006)** with a treatment duration of two to four weeks. Treatment can be discontinued after clinical recovery.

For moderate to severe infections, oral treatment with VGCV is the treatment of choice **(Anne-Laure, 2013).** International recommendations favor valganciclovir at a dosage of 900 mg twice a day, adapted to the patient's renal function. In addition, weekly biological monitoring is required to detect any toxicity of antiviral treatment as quickly as possible **(Kotton et al., 2013)**.

For any solid organ transplantation, it is recommended to continue treatment with IV GCV or oral VGCV until the following criteria are met: clinical resolution of symptoms, viremia below threshold values and at least two weeks of treatment **(Simon, 2014)**, as recurrence of CMV disease after treatment is possible, particularly after primary infection. Another important aspect of curative treatment is the reduction of immunosuppression **(Gargah et al., 2010).**

Diagnostic testing is an excellent tool for determining the duration of antiviral therapy for each patient. Patients with an undetectable CMV viral load at the end of therapy have a lower risk of recurrence than those whose viral load is still detectable **(Asberg et al., 2009).**

3.5.3 Follow-up on pathology

CMV infection or disease requires very regular follow-up:

3.5.3.1 Virological monitoring

Viral load represents the number of virus copies per milliliter of blood, and can be used to diagnose CMV infection, assess the efficacy of antiviral treatment or identify resistance to treatment.

The aim during treatment is to render the viral load undetectable, a sign of inhibited viral replication. This can be achieved by pp65 antigenemia, gene amplification or polymerase chain reaction (PCR).

Monitoring must be carried out on the same type of sample, using the same technique and in the same laboratory.

In the case of pre-emptive treatment, this follow-up should be weekly for at least 3 to 4 months after transplantation. The threshold beyond which treatment should be initiated should be defined following a clinical-biological discussion, depending on the PCR technique used and the patient's characteristics.

During antiviral treatment of the disease, viral load is monitored weekly. Discontinuation of treatment should be considered after two consecutive negative results at least one week apart **(Has, 2015).**

3.5.3.2 Biological monitoring

The drugs we use can cause toxicities that need to be controlled by regular biological monitoring:

With ganciclovir and valganciclovir, a blood count is recommended every day during initial treatment, then every 7 to 15 days during maintenance therapy. Creatinine clearance, a measure of glomerular filtration rate, should also be regularly monitored, so that dosage can be adjusted if renal function deteriorates.

With foscarnet, which carries a risk of nephrotoxicity and electrolyte disorders, creatinemia and calcemia should be monitored every 2 days during initial treatment, then once a week. Blood counts should be taken weekly during initial treatment and then twice a month. Kalemia and phosphatemia should also be monitored **(Vital et al., 2012).**

3.5.3.3 Immunological monitoring

Its purpose is to assess the patient's immune response by measuring HCMV-specific CD4+ and CD8+ T lymphocytes. Different. This follow-up is recommended to assess the risk of active CMV infection or disease. Most trials conducted are based on the detection of INFγ after stimulation of whole blood or peripheral mononuclear cells with CMV-specific antigens or peptides **(Kotton et al., 2013).**

The presence of sufficient numbers of T cells expressing cytokines such as INFγ, TNFα or IL2 is correlated with good CMV control in the short and long term. On the contrary, a lack of T cells is associated with an increased risk of viral replication **(Kumar et al., 2009; Lisboa et al., 2012; Widmann et al., 2008).**

Conclusion

Renal transplantation is the treatment of choice for chronic renal failure. However, it is fraught with complications, notably infectious, bacterial and viral, with cytomegalovirus infection at the top of the list. Cytomegalovirus is a serious, sometimes fatal viral infection with an unpredictable course.

The management of CMV infection in transplantation has evolved considerably in recent years, despite its high prevalence. The development of new-generation antivirals, the identification of risk factors, the determination of the serological status of the donor/recipient pair prior to transplantation, and the type of organ transplanted have all contributed to improved management of transplant patients. Standardization of laboratory tests, such as PCR, is essential for early treatment and follow-up.

In this study, we found that there was a close relationship between organ rejection and CMV infection, especially with increasing immunosuppressive therapy.

Prevention remains essential, with respect for operating time, monitoring of immunosuppressant toxicity and anti-infection prophylaxis, with the sole aim of preserving the graft and improving the graft recipient's quality of life.

The prospects are to envisage a retrospective multicenter study whose aim is to improve our knowledge of the frequency of CMV infection in the context of renal transplantation in Algeria and to minimize infectious complications, particularly opportunistic infections, through the development of new efficacious immunosuppressive molecules with fewer possible side effects.

References

-Abramovicz, D., Wissing, K., &Broeders, N. (2000). Immunosuppression strategies in renal transplantation at the beginning of the third millennium. *J Pharm Clin,* 32(4), 201-18.

- Agut, H. (2011). Herpesviruses and human herpesviroses. *Bull.Acad.Vét.France*, pp, 287-291.http://www.academie-veterinaire-defrance.org/

- Alain, S. & Mazeron, M. (2001). Cytomegalovirus infections. EMC 8-052-C-10. Inkinen, K., Soots, A., Krogerus, L., Loginov, R., Bruggeman, C., & Lautenschlager, I. (2005). Cytomegalovirus enhance expression of growth factors during the development of chronic allograft nephropathy in rats. *TranspIInt*, 18(6), 743-9.

- Alain, S., & Mazeron, M. (2003). Traité de virologie médicale. https://www.sfm-microbiologie.org/boutique/treatise-virologie-medicale/

- Alonso, A., & Oliver, J. (2004). Causes of death and mortality risk factors. Nephrol Dial Transplant ,19(3), 8-10.

- Anglicheau, D., Zuber, J., & Martinez, F. (2007) Kidney transplantation: performance and complications. *EMC Néphrologie*, pp.18-065-E-10
https://www.em- consulte.com/article/60959/renal-transplant-realization-and-completion

- Anne, S. & Victoria, M. (2019). Infectious complications after kidney transplantation. *Nephrology & Therapeutics*, 15(1), 37-42.

- Anne-Laure, F. (2013). *Incidence and risk factors for CMV resistance in a cohort of renal transplant patients* [Doctoral dissertation, University of Limoges]. Aurore.unilim.fr.
file:///C:/Users/USER/Downloads/M20133130.pdf

- Asberg, A., Humar, A., Jardine, A., Rollage, H., Pescovitz, M., Mouas, H., Bignamini, A., Toz, H., Dittmer, I., Montejo, M. & Hartmann, A. (2009). Long-termoutcomes of CMV diseasetreatmentwithvalganciclovir versus IV ganciclovir in solidorgan transplant recipients, *Am J Transplant,* 9(5), 1205-13.

- Asberg, A., Humar, A., Rollag, H., Jardine, A., Mouas, H., Pescovitz, M. et al. (2007). Oral Valganciclovir Is Noninferior to Intravenous Ganciclovir for the Treatment of Cytomegalovirus Disease in Solid Organ Transplant Recipients. *American journal of transplantation,* 7(9), 2106-2013.

- Audard, V., Baron, C., & Lang, P. (2005). Glomerulopathies and renal transplantation: de novo and recurrence. *EMC - Néphrologie*, 2(3), 125-137.

- Balssa, L., Bittard, H., & Kleinclauss, F. (2011). Immunosuppression in renal transplantation. *Progress in Urology*, 21, 250-3.
https://www.urofrance.org/base- bibliography/immunosuppression-in-transplantationrenale-0

- Barande, S. (2014). *Prevention and treatment of cytomegalovirus after transplantation.* [Doctoral dissertation, University of limoges].aurore.unilim.f
file:///C:/Users/pc/Downloads/P20143340.pdf

- Benjelloun, H., Laboudi, A., Marzouk, M.., Messnaoui, A., Rhou, H., & Balafrej, L. (2005). Conservative treatment of renal graft rupture. *Progrès en Urologie*, 15, 329-332.https://www.urofrance.org/base-bibliographique/traitement-conservateur-dune-rupture-dugreffon-renal

- Bernard, L. (2013). Physiology of the kidney and pathophysiological bases of renal diseases. Revue francophone des laboratoires. *Science direct,* (451), pp. 25-37.
https://www.sciencedirect.com/science/article/abs/pii/S1773035X13719932

- Biron, K. (2006). Antiviral drugs for cytomegalovirus diseases. *Antiviral research,* 71(2-3), 154-163.

- Boehme, K., Guerrero, M., & Compton, T. (2006). Human cytomegalovirus envelope glycoproteins B and H are necessary for TLR2 activation in permissive cells. *J ImmunolBaltimMd1950,* 177(10), 7094102-.

- Boppana, S., Rivera, L., Fowler, K., Mach, M., & Britt, W. (2001). Intrauterine Transmission of Cytomegalovirus to Infants of Women with Preconceptional Immunity. *N Engl J Med,* 344(18), 1366-71.

- -Bordage, M. (2015). *Devenir des patients de plus de 75 ans ayant une insuffisance rénale au stade 4* [Doctoral dissertation, University of Bejaïa].
www.univ bejaia.dz.http://www.univbejaia.dz/jspui/bitstream

- Bouabid, F., & Benamarr, L., et al. (2008). Profil épidémiologique donneurs vivants et transplantation rénale: communication libre; 10e réunion commune de la société Francophone de dialyse (SFD) Marrakech Palais des congrès Maroc, 26-29.

- Bresnahan, W. & Shenk, T. (2000). UL82 virion protein activates ex-pression of immediate early viral genes in human cytomegalovirus-infectedcells. *Proc. Natl. Acad. Sci. USA*, 97(26), 14506-14511.

- Bresnahan, W. & Shenk, T. (2000). A subset of viral transcripts packaged within human cytomegalovirus particles. *Science*, 288(5475), 2373-6.

- Brestrich, G., Zwinger, S., Fischer, A., Schmuck, M., Rohmhild, A., Hammer, M., Kurtz, A., Uharek, L., Knosalla, C., Lehmkuhl, H.,Volk, H., & Reinke, P. (2009). Adoptive T-cell therapy of lung transplanted patient with severe CMV disease and resistance to antiviral therapy. *Am j transplant,* 9(7), 1679-1684.
- Britt, W. & Boppana, S. (2004). Human cytomegalovirus virion proteins.Hum. *Immunol,* 65(5), 395-402.
- Britt, W. & Mach, M. (1996). Human cytomegalovirus glycoproteins. *Intervirology,* 39(5- 6), 40112-.
- Brown, N., Slater, D., Alvi, S., Elder, M., Sullivan, M., Bennett, P. (1999). Expression of 5- lipoxygenase and 5-lipoxygenase-activating protein in human fetal membranes throughout pregnancy and at term. *Mol Hum Reprod,* 5(7), 668-74.
- - Butcher, S.,Aitken, J., Mitchel, J., Gowen, B., & Dargan, D. (1998). Structure of the human cytomegalovirus B capsid by electron cryomicroscopy and image reconstruction. J StructBiol, 124(1), 70-6.
- Canaud, B., Ryckelynck, P., & Hourmant, Y. (2005). Nephrology-the replacement therapy of chronic end-stage renal disease. *La presse médicale,* 34(16), 1197-9.
- Cannon, M. & Davis, K. (2005).Washing our hands of the congenital cytomegalovirus disease epidemic. *BMC Public Health* 5, 70, 1471-2458. https://doi.org/10.1186/1471-2458-5-70
- Cannon, M., Schmid, D., & Hyde, T. (2010). Review of cytomegalovirus seroprevalance and demographic characteristics associated with infection. *Rev Med,* 20(4), 202 213.
- Cha, T., Tom, E., Kemble, G., Duke, G., Mocarski, E., & Spaete, R. (1996). Human cytomegalovirus clinical isolates carry at least 19 genes not found in laboratory strains. *J. Virol,* 70(1), 78-83.
- - Chan, G., Nogalski, M., &Yurochko, A. (2009). Activation of EGFR on monocytes is required for human cytomegalovirus entry and mediates cellular motility. *Proc NatlAcadSci U S A,* 106(52), 22369-22374.
- Cole, R. & Kuttner, A. (1926). A filtrable virus present in the submaxillary glands of guinea pigs. *J. Exp. Med*, 44, 855-873. https://www.ncbi.nlm.nih.gov/pmc/articles/PMC2131220/
- Compton, T., Kurt-Jones, E., Boehme, K., Belko, J., Latz, E., Golenbock, D., et al. (2003). Human cytomegalovirus activates inflammatory cytokine responses via CD14 and Toll like receptor 2. *J Virol*, 77(8), 458896-.

- - Compton, T., Nowlin, D. & Cooper, N. (1993). Initiation of human cytomegalovirus infection requires initial interaction with cell surface heparan sulfate. *Virology.avr*, 193(2), 83441-.

- Cook, C., Yenchar, J., Kraner, T., Davies, E., & Ferguson, R. (1998). Occult herpes family viruses may increase mortality in critically ill surgical patients. *Am J Surg*, 176(4), 357-360.

- Cotin, S. (2011). *Human cytomegalovirus, resistance mutations, and new antivirals.* [Doctoral dissertation, University of Limoges]. Aurore.unilim.fr. file:///C:/Users/pc/Downloads/2017LIMO0046.pdf

- Crough, T. & Khanna, R. (2009). Immunobiology of Human Cytomegalovirus: from Bench to Bed side. *Clin MicrobiolRev*, 22(1), 76-98.

- Crumpacker, C. (1992). Mechanism of action of foscarnet against viral polymerases. *Am J Med*, 92(2A), 3S-7S.

- Crumpacker, C. (1996). Ganciclovir. *N Engl j Med*, 335 (10), 335-721.

- Cui, X., Freed, D., Wang, D., Qiu, P., Li, F., Fu, T., Kauvar, L., & McVoy, M. (2017). Impact of Antibodies and Strain Polymorphisms on Cytomegalovirus Entry and Spread in Fibroblasts and Epithelial Cells, *J Virol*, 91(13), 1-17.

- Daroux, M., Gaxatte, C., Puisieux, F., Corman, B., & Boulanger, E. (2009). Renal aging: risk factors and nephroprotection. *Presse Med,* 38, 1667- 1679.https://coek.info/pdf-vieillissement-renal-facteurs-de-risque-et-nephroprotection-.html

- -Davison, A., Eberle, R., Ehlers, B., Hayward, G., Mcgeoch, D., Minson, A., Pellett, P., Roizman, B., Studdert, M.,&Thiry, E.(2009).The order Herpesvirales. *ArchVirol*, 154(1), 171-177.

- -Dennai, Y. (2012). *Prise en charge de l'insuffisance rénale chronique terminale en urgence (A propos de 140 cas).* [Doctor of Pharmacy thesis, Sidi Mohammed ben Abdallah University]. scolarite.fmp-usmba.ac.ma. http://scolarite.fmp-usmba.ac.ma/cdim/mediatheque/e_theses/9-12.pdf

- Descamps, V. (2014). *Cytomegalovirus infection* [Doctoral dissertation, University of Bordeaux]. Tel.archives-ouvertes.fr. https://dumas.ccsd.cnrs.fr/dumas-02328328

-Doublie, S., Sawaya, M., & Ellenberger, T. (1999). An open and closed case for all polymerases. *Structure*, 7(4), 31-35.

- -Dussol, B. (2011). Different stages of chronic renal failure: recommendations. Immunoanalysis and specialized biology. *Revues générales et analyses prospectives*, 26, 55-59.https://sci-hub.tw/10.1016/j.immbio.2010.12.003

- Eddleston, M., Peacock, S., Juniper, M., & Warrell, D. (1997). Severe Cytomegalovirus Infection in Immunocompetent Patients. *Clinical Infectious Diseases*, 24(1), 52-56.

- Einsele, H.,Roosnek, E., Rufer, N., Sinzger, C., Riegler, S., Löffler, J., Grigoleit, U. et al. (2002). Infusion of cytomegalovirus (CMV)-specific T cells for the treatment of CMV infection not responding to antiviral chemotherapy. *Blood,* 99(11), 3916-22.

- Esclatine, A., & Géniteau-Legendre, M. (2002). Human cytomegalovirus and intestinal epithelial cells. 6(4), 276-277.

- -Fabien, B. (2015). Adoptive immunotherapy after stem cell allograft: interest and production of anti-cmv T lymphocytes [PhD thesis, Université de Mantes]. pdfs.semanticscholar.org.
file:///C:/Users/pc/Downloads/breletPH15.pdf

- Fakhfkh H., H.S., Hachicha J, (2006). Renal transplantation from living related donor. A propos de 95 cas. Service d'Urologie Sfax, Tunisia. Communication (PA43) 6e congrès de la Société francophone de transplantation, 6-9.

- Feire, A., Roy, R., Manley, K., & Compton, T. (2010). The glycoprotein B disintegrin like domainbinds beta 1 integrin to mediate cytomegalovirus entry. *J Virol,* 84(19), 10026-37.

- Fietze, E., Prösch, S., Reinke, P., Stein, J., Döcke, WD., Staffa, G. et al. (1994).Cytomegalovirus infection in transplant recipients.The role of tumor necrosis factor. *Transplantation,* 58(6), 675-680.

- Fishman, J., (2007). Infection in solid-organ transplant recipients. *N Engl J Med*, 357(25), 2601-2614.

- Gael, C. (2006). *Human cytomegalovirus and antivirals: genetic supports of resistance and targets of new antivirals* [PhD thesis, Université de limoges]. Aurore.unilim.fr. C:/Users/USER/Downloads/2006LIMO0013%20(1).pdf

- Gamadia, L., Remmerswaal, E., Weel, J., Bemelman, F., van Lier, R. et al. (2003). Primary immune responses to human CMV: a critical role for IFN-gamma-producing CD4+ T cells in protection against CMV disease. *Blood,* 101(7), 2686-2692.

- Gandhi, M. & Khanna, R. (2004). Human cytomegalovirus: clinical aspects, immune regulation, and emerging treatments. *Lancet Infect Dis*, 4(12), 725-38.

- Gargah, A., Labassi, M., & Lakhoua,R. (2010). Cytomegalovirus infections after renal transplantation: experience from a pediatric nephrology center. *Revue Tunisienne d'Infectiologie*, 4, 23-26.
https://www.infectiologie.org.tn/pdf_ppt_docs/revues/1-2010/infections_cytomega.pdf

- Gargah, T., Labassi, A., & Lakhoua, M. (2010). Cytomegalovirus infections followingrenal transplantation: the experience of a paediatric center. *Tunisienne d'Infectiologie*, 4(3), 23 - 26.

- Gaston, R., & Cosio, F. (2004). Transplantation in the diabetic patient with advanced chronic kidney disease: a task force report. *Am J Kidney Dis,* 44(3), 529-542.

- Gerna, G., Revello, M., Baldanti, F., Percivalle, E., & Lilleri, D. (2017). The pentamericcomplex of humanCytomegalovirus: celltropism, virus dissemination, immune response and vaccine development. *J GenVirol,* 98, 2215 2234. https://pubmed.ncbi.nlm.nih.gov/28809151/

- Ghods, A. (2007). Organ Transplantation in Iran. *Saudi J Kidney Transplant.* 185(4), 648-655.

- Gibson, W. (1996). Structure and assembly of the virion. *Intervirology,* 39(5-6), 389-400.

- Gicklhorn, D., Markus, E., Grit, M., Mats, O., & Klaus, R. (2003). Differential effects of glycoprotein B epitope-specific antibodies on human cytomegalovirus-induced cell-cell fusion. *J GenVirol,* 84(7), 1859-62.

- Gore, J., pham, P., Danovitch, G. et al. 2006. Obesity and outcome following renal Transplantation. *Am J Transplant*, 6(2), 357-363.

- Gratacap-Cavallier, B., Morand, P., Benbassa, A., Micoud, M., Seigneurin, J., Dutertre, N., Bosson, J. et al. (1998). Cytomegalovirus infection in pregnant women. Prospective sero-epidemiological study of 1018 women in Isère. *J. Gynecol. Obstet. Biol. Reprod*, 27(2), 161-6.

- Greijer, A., Dekkers, C.,& Middeldorp, G. (2000). Human cytomegalovirus virions differentially incorporate viral and host cell RNA during the assemblyprocess. *J Virol,* 74(19), 9078-82.

- Gretchen, L., Bentz, & Yurochko, A. (2008). Human CMV infection of endothelial cells induces an angiogenic response through viral binding to EGF receptor and β1 and β3 integrins, 105(14), 5531-5536.

- -Gueutin, V. (2012). Renal physiology. *Cancer Bulletin*, (99), pp. 237-249. https://doi.org/10.1684/bdc.2011.1482

- Guyton C. (1998). A treatise on physiology. [E-book].

- Halloran, P. (2004). Immunosuppressive drugs for kidney transplantation. *N Engl J Med,* 351(26), 2715-29.

- Hantz, S., Mazeron, M., Alain, S. & Leruez-ville, M. (2009). Treatment of cytomegalovirus hmain (CMV) infections. Médecine thérapeutique, 15, 221-222. https://hal-unilim.archives-ouvertes.fr/hal-00535739

- Hariharan, S., McBride, M., & Cohen, E. (2003). Evolution of endpoints for renal transplant outcome. *Am J Transplant*, 8, 933-41.https://onlinelibrary.wiley.com/doi/full/10.1034/j.1600-6143.2003.00176.x

- Harwardt, T., Lukas, S., Zenger, M., Reitberger, T., Danzer, D., Ubner, T., Munday, D.,Nevels, M., & Paulus, C. (2016). Human Cytomegalovirus Immediate-Early 1 Protein Rewires Upstream STAT3 to Downstream STAT1 Signaling Switching an IL6-Type to an IFNγLike Response. *PLos Pathog*, 12(7), e1005748.

- Has. (2015). Evaluation of cytomegalovirus viral load measurement by gene amplification in allograft recipients. www.has-sante.fr. http://www.hassante.fr/portail/upload/docs/application/pdf/201508/argumentaire_cmv_vd.pdf

- Henell K.R, Chou S., Norman DJ. (1989). Use of cytomegalovirus-seropositive donor kidneys in seronegative patients: results of prospective serotesting and matching in one center. *Transplant Proc*, 21(1), 2082-3.

- Hirsch, H., Lautenschlager, I., Pinsky, B., et al. (2013). An international multicenter performance analysis of cytomegalovirus load tests. *Clin Infect Dis*, 56, 367-73. https://academic.oup.com/cid/article/56/3/367/429148

- -Hitchcock, M., Jaffe, H., Martin, J., & Stagg, R. (1996). Cidofovir, a new agent with potent anti-herpesvirus activity. *AntivirChemChemother*, 7, 115-27.

- -Hricik, D., O'Toole, M., Schulak, J., & Herson, J. (1993). Steroiden -Free Immunodepression in cyclosporine treated renal transplant recipients: a meta analysis. *J AM. Soc Nephrol*, 4(6), 1300-1305.

- Humar, A. & Snydman, D. (2009). Cytomegalovirus in solidorgan transplant recipients. *Am J Transplant*, 4(8), 78-86.

- Humar, A., & Michaels, M. (2006). American Society of Transplantation recommendations for screening, monitoring and reporting of infectious complications in immunosuppression trials in recipients of organ transplantation. *Am J Transplant,* 6(2), 262-274.

- Humar, A., Gregson, D., Caliendo, A., McGeer, A., Malkan, G., krajden, M., Corey, P., Greig, P., walmsley, S., Levy, G. & Mazzulli, T. (1999). Clinical utility of quantitative cytomegalovirus viral loaddetermination for predictingcytomegalovirusdisease in liver transplant recipients. *Transplantation*, 68(9), 1305-11.

- Humar, A., Mazzulli, T., Moussa, G., Razonable, R., Paya, CV., Pescovitz, M., Covington, E., & Alecock, E. (2005). Clinical utility of cytomegalovirus (CMV) serology testing in high-risk CMV D+/R- transplant recipients. *Am J Transplant*, 5(5), 1065-1070.

- Imbert, B. (2002). Epidemiology of cytomegalovirus infections (Edition Scientifique et médicales). [E-book]. Elsevier. Paris

- Irmiere, A. & Gibson, W. (1983). Isolation and characterization of a noninfectious virion-like particle released from cells infected with human strains of cytomegalovirus. *Virology*, 130(1), 118-33.

- Jaboulay, M., et al (1896). Experimental research on arterial suturing and grafting. *Lyon Med,* 8, 81-97.

- Jabs, D., Enger, C., Forman, M., & Dunn, J. (1998). Incidence of foscarnet resistance and cidofovir resistance in patients treated for cytomegalovirus retinitis. *Antimicrob Agents Chemother*, 42(9), 2240-2244.

- Jacobson, M., & Mark, A. (1997). Treatment of cytomegalovirus retinis in patients with the acquiered immunodeficiency syndrome. *N. Engl. J. Med*, 337(9), 105-114.

- Jesionek, A. & Kiolemenoglou, B. (1904). Ubereinenbefund von protozoer nartigen gebilden in den organeneinesheriditar -luetishenfotus. *Munch.Med.Wochenschr*, 51, 1905-1907.

- Johann, S. , Runhild, L., & Christophe, P. (2013). The human body anatomy and physiology 635 illustrations. Lacour, B. (2013). Physiology of the kidney and pathophysiological bases of renal diseases. *Revue francophone des laboratoires,* 2013(451), 25-37.

- Julie, D. (2015). *Congenital cytomegalovirus infection: evaluation of the prevalence of vestibular damage* [Doctoral dissertation, University of Toulouse III-Paul Sabatier]. thesesante.ups-tlse.fr.
http://thesesante.ups-tlse.fr.http://thesesante.ups-tlse.fr/1055/1/2015TOU31552.pdf

- Kabore, R. (2017). *Prediction of graft loss in young kidney transplant patients.* [Doctoral dissertation, Université De Bordeaux], thèsestel.archives-ouvertes.fr. https://tel.archives-ouvertes.fr/tel-01685558/document

- Kamar, N., Mengelle, C., & Rostaing, L. (2007). Alteration of direct and indirect effects of cytomegalovirus. *Exp Clin Transplant*, 5(2), 727-30.

- Kamar, N., Mengelle, C., Esposito, L., Guitard, J., Mehrenberger, M., Lavayssière, L. et al. (2008). Predictive factors for cytomegalovirus reactivation in cytomegalovirus-seropositive kidney-transplant patients. *J Med Virol,* 80(6):10121017.

- Kapranos, N., Petrakou, E., Anastasiadou, C., & Kotronias, D. (2003). Detection of herpes simplex virus, cytomegalovirus, and Epstein-Barr virus in the semen of men attending an infertilityclinic. *Fertility and sterility*, 79(3), 156-670.

- Kdigo (2009). Clinical practice guideline for the care of kidney transplant recipients. Am J Transplant,. 9: p. S1-S155. https://pubmed.ncbi.nlm.nih.gov/19845597/

- Klemola, E. & Kaarianinen, L. (1965). Cytomegalovirus as a possible cause of a disease resembling infectious mononucleosis.*Br Med J*, 2(5470), 1099-1102.

- Knoll, G. (2013). Kidney transplantation in the older adult. *Am J Kidney Dis*, 61(5), 7907.

- Kotton, C., Kumar, D., Caliendo, A., Asberg, A., Chou, S., Danziger-Isakov, L., & Humar, A. (2013). Updated International Consensus Guidelines on the Management of Cytomegalovirus in Solid-Organ Transplantation. *Transplantation,* 96(4), 333-60.

- Kotton, C., kumar, D., Caliendo, A., Asberg, A., Chou, S., Snydman, D., Allen, U.& Humar, A. (2010). International consensus guidelines on the management of cytomegalovirus in solidorgantranspkantation. *Transplantation,* 89(7), 779-95.

- Kumar, D., Chernenko, S., Moussa, G., Cobos, I., Manuel, O., Preiksaitis, J., Venkataraman, S. & Humar, A. (2009). Cell-mediated immunity to predict cytomegalovirus disease in high-risk solid organ transplant recipients. *American Journal of Transplantation*, 9(5), 121- 422.

- Kurath, S. & Rech, B. (2010). Cytomegalovirus and transmission via breastmilk: how to support breastmilk to premature infants and prevent severe infection. *Infect Dis J*, 29(7), 680-1.

- Lacombe, M. (2002). La transplantation rénale, une épopée centenaire Renal transplantation, a hundred-year old adventure. *Annales de Chirurgie*, 127(7), 542-548.

- Lammers, C., Schweitzer, P., Facchinetti, P., Arrang, J., Madamba, S.,Siggins, G., et al. (1996). Arachidonate 5-lipoxygenase and its activating protein: prominent hippocampal expression and role in somatostatin signaling. *J Neurochem*, 66(1), 147-52.

- Lay, L., Xu, Z., Zhou, J., Lee, k. & Amidon, G. (2008). Molecular basis of prodrug activation by humanvalacyclovirase, an a-aminoacid ester hydrolase. *J BiolChem*, 283(14), 9381-9327.

- Lebranchu, Y. (1997). Aspect épidémiologique et immunologique; Principes de traitement et surveillance, complication et pronostic de la transplantation d'organes. *Revue du praticien N° spécial " prélèvement et greffe ".*

- Legendre, C., Loupy, A, Anglicheau A, et al. (2010). Humoral acute rejection. [E-book]. Paris: Elsevier Masson.

- Legendre, C., & coll. (2012). Renal transplantation, (Lavoisier edition). [E-book].

- Lehner, R., Meyer, H., & Mach, M. (1989). Identification and characterization of a human cytomegalovirus gene coding for a membrane protein that is conserved among human herpesviruses. *J Virol*, 63(9), 3792-800.

- Leruez-Ville, M. (2001). Le diagnostic virologique de l'infection à cytomégalovirus humain". Médecine thérapeutique [Doctoral thesis, University of Limoges]. aurore.unilim.fr. file:///C:/Users/DELL-10/AppData/Local/Temp/P20143340.pdf

- Ligat, G. (2017). *Human cytomegalovirus, resistance mutations, and new therapeutic targets.* [Doctoral dissertation, University of Limoges]. Aurore.unilim.fr. file:///C:/Users/USER/Downloads/2017LIMO0046.pdf

- Lisboa, LF., Kumar, D., Wilson, LE. &Humar, A. (2012).Clinical utility of cytomegalovirus cell-mediated immunity in transplant recipients with cytomegalovirus viremia.*Transplantation,* 93(2), 195-200.

- Littler, E., Stuart, A. & Chee, M. (1992). Human cytomegalovirus UL97 open rading frame encodes a protein that phosphorylates the antiviral nucleoside analogue ganciclovir. *Nature,* 358(6382), 160-162.

- Liu, B. & Stinski, M. (1992). Human cytomegalovirus contains a tegument protein that enhances transcription from promoters with upstream ATF and AP-1 cis-acting elements. *J Virol,* 66(7), 4434-44.

- Lopez, C., Richard, L., Simmons, R., Mauer, M., John S.Najarian, J., & Robert, A., Good, R. (1974). Association of renal allograft rejection with virus infections. *American Journal Of Medicine*, 56(9), 280-289.

- Lowance, D., Neumayer, H., Legendre, C., Squifflet, J., Kovarik, J., Brennan, P., Norman, D.,& Lucie, M. (2013). *Study models of new anti-CMV molecules in the placenta.* [PhD thesis, Université De Limoges]. aurore.unilim.fr. file:///C:/Users/pc/Downloads/2013LIMO310D.pdf

- Lucie, M. (2013). Study models of new anti-CMV molecules in the placenta. [PhD thesis, University of Limoges]. *aurore.unilim.fr.* file:///C:/Users/DELL-10/AppData/Local/Temp/2013LIMO310D.pdf

- Ludwig, A. & Hengel, H. (2009). Epidemiological impact and disease burden of congenital cytomegalovirus infection in Europe. *Eurosurveillance*, 14(9).

- Macagno, A., Bernasconi, N., Vanzetta, F., Dander, E., Sarasini, A., Revello, M., Gerna, G., Sallusto, F., & Lanzavecchia, A. (2010). Isolation of Human Monoclonal Antibodies That Potently Neutralize Human Cytomegalovirus Infection by Targeting Different Epitopes on the gH/gL/UL128-131A Complex. *J. Virol.* 84(2), 1005-1013.

- Mamzer-Bruneel, M. (2008). Infections in renal transplant patients, excluding viral infections. *Actualités néphrologiques Jean Hamburger*, pp 59- 73 .https://pascalfrancis.inist.fr/vibad/index.php?action=getRecordDetail&idt=20870480

- Man, N., Touam, M., & Jungers, P. (2010). L'Hémodialyse de suppléance; (Médecine Sciences). [E-book]. Flammarion.

- Martinez-Martin, N., Marcandalli, J., Huang, C., Arthur, C., Perotti, M., Foglierini, M., Ho, H., Dosey, A., Shriver, S., Payandeh, J., et al. (2018). An Unbiased Screen for Human Cytomegalovirus Identifies Neuropilin-2 as a Central Viral Receptor. *Cell,* 174(5), 1158- 1171.

- Matthews, T. & Boehme, R. (1988). Antiviral activity and mechanism of action ganciclovir. *Rev infect Dis*, 10, 490-494. https://pubmed.ncbi.nih.gov/2847285/

- Maude, R. (2016). *Pathophysiology of cytomegalovirus infection on human neural progenitors* [PhD thesis, Université Paul Sabatier - Toulouse III]. tel.archives-ouvertes.fr .https://tel.archives-ouvertes.fr/tel-01635355/document

- Mendez, R., Keating, M., Coggon, G., Crips, A., & Lee, I. (1999). Valacyclovir for the prevention of cytomegalovirus disease after renal transplantation. International Valacyclovir Cytomegalovirus Prophylaxis Transplantation Study Group. *N Engl J Med*, 340(19), 1462-1470.

- Metselaar, H., & W. Weinarn, W. (1989). Cytomegalovirus infection and renal transplantation. *J. Antimicrob. Chemother.* 23(10), 37-47.

- Meyer-König, U., Ebert, K., Schrage, B.,Pollak, S.,& Hufert, F. (1998). Simultaneous infection of healthy people with multiple human cytomegalovirus strains. *The Lancet,* 352(9136), 1280-1281.

- Mocarski, J. (2001). Cytomegaloviruses and Their Replication. In Knipe D, Howley P (ed), Fields virology (Lippincott Williams and Wilkins). [E-book]. Philadelphia. https://www.researchgate.net/publication/239490323

- Mombazet, A. (2010). *Le pharmacien d'officine face au patient dialysé Réalisation d'un outil de formation destiné à l'équipe officinale* [Doctoral thesis in pharmacy, Université Henri Poincare-Nancé]. hal.univ-lorraine.fr. https://hal.univ-lorraine.fr/hal-01738871/document

- Moulin, B. & Peraldi, M. (2014). Nephrology. (Universitaire des enseignants de néphrologie) (France). [E-book]. Paris: Ellipses.

-Moulin, B., & Peraldi, M. (2016). Nephrology. [E-book]. France: ECN

- Sayegh, M., & Carpenter, C. (2004). Transplantation 50 years later: progress, challenges, and promises. *N Engl J Med*, 351(26), 2761-6.

- Mourad G., Garrigue V., Bismuth J., Szwarc I., Delmas S., Iborra F. (2005). Follow-up and non-immunological complications of renal transplantation. *EMC (Elsevier SAS, Paris), Néphrologie,* 2(2), 61-82.

- Mourad, G., Garrigue, V., Delmas, S., Szwarc, I., Deleuze, S., Bismuth, J., Bismuth, M., & Secondy, M. (2005). Infectious and neoplastic complications after renal transplantation. *EMC-Néphrologie*, 2(4), 158-181.

- Mourad, G., Rostaing, L., Legendre, C., Garrigue, V., Thervet, E., & Durand, D. (2004). Sequential protocols using basiliximab versus antithymocyte globulins in renal-transplant patients receiving mycophenolatemofetil and steroids. *Transplantation*, 78(4), 584590.

- Muriel, F. (2010). *Human cytomegalovirus: variability, recombination and pUL40 protein* [Doctoral dissertation, Université Victor Segalen Bordeaux 2]. www.theses.fr. file:///C:/Users/pc/Downloads/Faure_-_Muriel_-_these_et_annexes%20(2).pdf

- Pang, X., Fox, J., Fenton, J., et al. (2009). Inter laboratory comparison of cytomegalovirus viral loads assays. *Am J Transplant*, 9, 258-68. https://onlinelibrary.wiley.com/doi/full/10.1111/j.1600-6143.2008.02513.x

- Paoletti , E., Amidone , M., Massarino , F., & Cannella, G. (2009). Association of arterial hypertension with renal target organ damage in kidney transplant recipients: the predictive role of ambulatory blood pressure monitoring. *Transplantation,* 87(12), 1864-1869.

- Pass, R. (2004). Cytomegalovirus. Fields BN, Knipe DM eds. *Virology:* Raven Press, NewYork, 2, 2675-2705.

- Patel, R., & Paya, C., (1997). Infections in solid-organ transplant recipients. *ClinMicrobiol Rev,* 10(1), 86-124.

- - Paulus, C., & Nevels, M. (2009). The Human Cytomegalovirus Major Immediate Early Proteins as Antagonists of Intrinsic and Innate Antiviral Host Responses. *Viruses,* 1(3), 760-779.

- Paya, C., Humar, A., Dominguez, E., Washburn, K., Blumberg, E., Alexander, B., Freeman, R., Heaton, N., & Pescovitz, M. (2004). Valganciclovir Solid Organ Transplant Study Group. Efficacy and safety of valganciclovir vs. oral ganciclovir for prevention of cytomegalovirus disease in solid organ transplant recipients. *Am J Transplant*, 4(4), 611-620.

- Perrottet, N., Decosterd, A., Meylan, P., Pascual,M., Biollaz, j. & Buclin, T. (2009). Valganciclovir in adult solid organ transplant recipients: pharmacokinetic and pharmacodynamics characteristics and clinical interpretation of plasma concentration measurements. *Clin pharmacokinet*, 48(6), 399-418.

- Petitclerc, T. (1998). Hemodialysis: general principles and treatment modalities. *Médecine thérapeutique*, 2(7), 557-66.

- Pierre, B. (2012). *Pharmaceutical treatment of cytomegalovirus (CMV) infections with ganciclovir: exploratory study in renal transplantation* [Doctoral dissertation, University of Limoges]. Aurore.unilim.fr. C:/Users/USER/Downloads/P20143340%20(2).pdf

- Razonable, R., & Hayden, R. (2013). Clinical utility of viral load in management of cytomegalovirus infection after solid organ transplantation. *Clin Microbiol Rev*, 26, 703-27. https://cmr.asm.org/content/26/4/703.short

- Reichenberger, F., Dickenmann, M., Binet, I., Soler, M., Bolliger, C., Steiger, J., et al. (2001). Diagnostic yield of bronchoalveolar lavage following renal transplantation. *Transpl Infect Dis*, 3(1), 2-7.

- Remuzzi, G., Grinyo, J., Ruggenenti, P., Beatini, M., et al. (1999). Early experience with dual kidney transplantation in adults using expanded donor criteria. J Am Soc Nephrol, 10(12) 259 -8.

- Reusser, P. (1996). Herpes virus resistance to antiviral drugs: are view of the mechanisms, clinical importance and therapeutic options. *J hosp infect*, 33(4), 235-48.

- Reynolds, D., Stagno, S., Hosty, T., Tiller, M., & Alford, C. (1973). Maternal cytomegalovirus excretion and perinatal infection. *The New England journal of medicine,* 289(1), 1-5.

- Roche. RCP Cymevan. 2014.

- Rodriguez, A., Park, H., Mao, C., & Beese, L. (2000). Crystal structure of a pol alpha family DNA polymerase from the hyper thermophili carchaeon Thermococcus sp. *9 degrees N-7. J MolBiol,* 299(2), 447-462.

- Rowshani, A., Bemelman, F., Leeuwen, E., Lier, R., & Berge, I. (2005). Clinical and immunologic aspects of cytomegalovirus infection in solid organ transplant recipients.*Transplantation*, 79(4), 381-386.

- Rubin, M. (2011). Hypertension Following Kidney Transplantation. *Chronic Kidney Disease,* 18(1), 17-22.

- Ruellan-Euqene, G., Barjot, P., Campet, M., & vabret, A. et al. (1996). Evaluation of viralogica 1 procedures ta detect fetal human cytomegalovirus infection: avidity of IgG antibodies, virus detection in amniotic fluid and maternai serum. *J. Med. Viral*, 50(1), 9-15.

- Sagedal, S., Nordal, K., Hartmann A. Sund, S., Scott, H., Degré, M., Foss, A., Leivestad, T., Osnes, K., Fauchald, P., & Rollag, H. (2002). The impact of cytomegalovirus infection and disease on rejection episodes in renal allograft recipients. *Am J Transplant*, 2(9), 850-6.

- Sagedal, S., Nordal, K., Hartmann, A., Degré, M., Holter, E., Foss, A., et al. (2000). A prospective study of the natural course of cytomegalovirus infection and disease in renal allograft recipients,*Transplantation*, 70(8), 1166-1174.

- Salvadori, M., Rosati, A., Di Maria, L., Becherelli, P., Moscarelli, L., Bandini, S., Piperno, R., Larti, A., Gallo, M. & Bertoni, E. (2005). Immunosuppression in renal transplantation: Viral diseases and chronic allograft nephropathy. *Transplant Proc*, 37(6), 2500-1.

- Sanchez, V., Clark, C., Yen, J., Dwarakanath, R., & Spector, D. (2002). Viable human cytomegalovirus recombinant virus with an internaldeletion of the IE2 86 gene affects late stages of viral replication. *J Virol*, 76(6), 2973-89.

- Sathiyamoorthy, K., Chen, J., Longnecker, R., & Jardetzky, T. (2017). The Complexity in herpesvirus entry. *CurrOpinVirol*, 24, 97-104. https://pubmed.ncbi.nlm.nih.gov/28538165/

- Schulak, J., Hricik, D., Toole, M., & Herson, J. (1993). Steroid-free immunosuppression in cyclosporine-treated renal transplant recipients: a meta-analysis. *Journal of the American society of nephrology*, 4(6), 1300-1305.https://jasn.asnjournals.org/content/4/6/1300.short

- Segondy, M. (2009). Human cytomegalovirus Encycl. Biologie Médicale. Anglicheau, D., Martinez, F., Méjean, A, et al. (2007). Renal transplantation: performance and complications. (EMC Néphrologie). [E-book]. Paris: Elsevier Masson.

- Sherwood (2006). Human physiology. [E-book].

- Sijmons, S., Van Ranst, M., & Maes, P. (2014). Genomic and functional characteristic of human cytomegalovirus revealed by next-generation sequencing.*Viruses*, 6(3), 1049-1072.

- Simon, B. (2014). *Prevention and treatment of cytomegalovirus after transplantation* [Doctoral dissertation, University of Limoges].Aurore.unilim.fr. file:///C:/Users/USER/Downloads/P20143340%20(7).pdf

- Simpson, J., Chow, J., Baker, J., Avdalovic, N., Yuan, S., Au, D., Co, M.S., Vasquez, M., Britt,W., & Coelingh, K. (1993). Neutralizing monoclonal antibodies that distinguish three antigenic sites on human cytomegalovirus glycoprotein H have conformationally distinct binding sites. *J Virol*, 67(1), 489-496.

- Sinclair, J.,& Sissons, P. (2006). Latency and reactivation of human cytomegalovirus. *Journal of General Virology*, 87(7), 1763-79.

- Sinzger, C., Grefte, A., Bodo, P., Annette, S., .Hauw, T. & Gerhar, D. (1995). Fibroblasts, epithelial cells, endothelial cells and smooth muscle cells are major targets of human cytomegalovirus infection in lung and gastrointestinal tissues, 76(4).

- Smith, M. (1956).Propagation in Tissue Cultures of a Cytopathogenic Virus from Human Salivary Gland Virus (SGV) Disease. *ExpBiol* Med, 92(2), 424-430.

- Söderberg-Nauclér, C., Fish, K., & Nelson, J. (1997). Reactivation of latent human cytomegalovirus by allogeneic stimulation of blood cells from healthy donors. *Cell,* 91(1), 119-126.

- Soroceanu, L., Akhavan, A., & Cobbs, C. (2008). Platelet-derived growth factor-alpha receptor activation is required for human cytomegalovirus infection. *Nature,* 455(7211), 391-5.

- Streblow, D., Varnum, S., Smith, R., & Nelson, A. (2006). A proteomics analysis of Human Cytomegalovirus particles. Cytomegalovirus, molecular biology and immunology Chapter. 5, 91-110. https://www.caister.com/hsp/abstracts/cmv/05.html

- Sumitran-Holgersson, S. (2001). HLA-specific alloantibodies and renal graft outcome. *Nephrology Dialysis Transplantation,* 16(5), 897-904.

- Tabeta, K., Georgel, P., Janssen, E., Du, X., Hoebe, K., & Crozat, K. (2004). Toll-like receptors 9 and 3 as essential components of innate immune defense against mouse cytomegalovirus infection. *Proc Natl AcadSci U S A,* 101(10), 3516 21.

- Tomtishen III, J. (2012). Human cytomegalovirus tegument proteins (pp65, pp71, pp150, pp28). *Virol J,* 9, 22-28 https://pubmed.ncbi.nlm.nih.gov/22251420/

- Torres-Madriz, G. & Boucher, H. (2008). Immunocompromised hosts: perspectives in the treatment and prophylaxis of cytomegalovirus disease in solid-organ transplant recipients. *Clin Infect Dis,* 47(5), 702-11.

- Tortora & Grabowski (2001). Principle of anatomy and physiology. [E-book].

- Tortora. G., and Angostakos N P. (1988). principle of anatomy and physiology. [E-book].

- Tu, W., Chen, S., Sharp, M., Dekker, C., Manganello, M. Eileen, C., Tongson, Holden, T., Maecker, Tyson, H. et al. (2004). Persistent and selective deficiency of CD4+ T cell immunity to cytomegalovirus in immunocompetent young children. *JImmunol,* 172(5), 3260- 7.

- Valiquette, L. & Quérin, S. (2000). Physiology of kidney and urinary tract diseases. [Ebook].

- Vanarsdall, A., & Johnson, D. (2012). Human cytomegalovirus entry in to cells. *CurrOpinVirol,* 2(1), 37-42.

- Vanarsdall, A., Howard, P., Wisner, T., & Jonhson, D. (2016). Human Cytomegalovirus gH/gL Forms a Stable Complex with the Fusion Proteing B in Virions. *PLoSPathog,* 12(4), e1005564.

- Venema, H., van den Berg, AP., van Zanten, C., van Son, W., van der Giessen, M., & TH, T. (1994). Natural killer cell responses in renal transplant patients with cytomegalovirus infection. *J Med Virol,* 42(2), 188-92.

- Vigneau, C., Fulgencio, J., Vincent, F., Tchala, K., & Rondeau, E. (2001). Existe-t-il un âge limite pour le don d'organes, Service de néphrologie Transplantation hôpital Tenon Paris. *Ann. Fr. Anaesth. Rea*, 20(8), 723-726.
- Vincent, B. & Pierre, Y. (2006). Chronic renal failure: management. *Forum Med suisse, curriculum,* 6(36), 794-803.
- Vital, D., Le Jeunne C. Dorosz. (2012). Guide pratique des médicaments. Maloine. Kotton, C., Kumar, D., Caliendo, A., Asberg, A., Chou, S., Danziger-Isakov, L. & Humar, A. (2013). CMV Consensus Group International Transplantation Society. Updated international consensus guidelines on the management of cytomegalovirus in solid-organ transplantation. *Transplantation,* 96(4), 333-60.
- Vivier, E., Tomasello, E., Baratin, M., Walzer, T., & Ugolini, S. (2008). Functions of natural killer cells. *Nat Immunol*, 9(5), 50310-.
- Wagstaff, A., & Bryson. H. (1994). Foscarnet. A reappraisal of its antiviral activity, pharmacokinetic properties and therapeutic use in immunocompromised patients with viral infections. *Drugs,* 48(2), 199-226.
- Wang, X., Huang, D., Huong, S., & Huang, E. (2005). Integrin alphavbeta3 is a co-receptor for human cytomegalovirus. *Nat Med,* 11(5), 515-521.
- Wang, Z., La Rosa, C., Mekhoubad, S.,Lacey, F.,Villacres, M., Markel, S., Longmate, J., Ellenhorn, I., Siliciano, F., Buck, C.,Britt, W., & Diamond, D. (2004). Attenuatedpoxvirusesgenerateclinically relevant frequencies of CMV-specific T cells. *Blood,* 104(3), 847-856.
- Wéclawiak, H., Kamar, N., Mengelle, C., Guitard, J., Esposito, L., Lavayssière, L. et al. (2008). Cytomegalovirus prophylaxis with valganciclovir in cytomegalovirus-seropositive kidneytransplant patients. *J Med Virol*, 80(7), 1228-1232.
- Weclawiak, H., Mengelle, C., Ould Mohamed, A., Izopet, J., Rostaing, L., & Kamar, N. (2010). Effect of cytomegalovirus in transplantation and place of antiviral prophylaxis. *Nephrology & Therapeutics,* 6(6), 505-512.
- Weller, T. (1970). Cytomegaloviruses: the difficult years. *J Infect Dis,* 122(6), 5329-5450.
- Widmann, T., Sester, U., Gärtner, B., Schubert, J., Pfreundschuh, M., Köhler, H., & Sester, M. (2008). Levels of CMV specific CD4 T cells are dynamic and correlate with CMV viremia after allogeneic stem cell transplantation. *PloS one,* 3(11), 36-34.
- Wiesner, R., Marin, E., Porayko, M., Steers, J., Krom, R., Paya, C. (1993). Advances in the diagnosis, treatment, and prevention of cytomegalovirus infections after liver transplantation Gastroenterol. *Clin.North.Am,* 22(15), 351-366.

- Williame, A. (2019). *The challenge of congenital cytomegalovirus infection.* [Doctoral dissertation, University of Geneva]. archive-ouverte.unige.ch. https://archive-ouverte.unige.ch/unige:128065

- Wright, L., Tuder, R., Wang, J., Cool, C., Lepley, R., Voelkel, N. (1998). 5 Lipoxygenase and 5-lipoxygenase activating protein (FLAP) immunoreactivity in lungs from patients with primary pulmonary hypertension. *Am J RespirCrit Care Med*, 157(1), 219-29.

- Wu, Y., Prager, A., Boos, S., Resch, M., Brizic, I., Mach, M., Wildner, S., Scrivano, L., & Adler, B. (2017). Human cytomegalovirus glycoprotein complex gH/gL/gO uses PDGFR-α as akey for entry, *PLoSPathog,* 13(4), e1006281.

- Yeung, J., Tong, K., & Chan H. (1998). Clinical pattern, risk factors, and outcome of CMV infection in renal transplant recipients: local experience. Transplant Proc, 30, 3144-5. https://d1wqtxts1xzle7.cloudfront.net/

- Yu, X., Trang, P., Shah,S., et al. (2005). Dissecting human cytomegalovirus gene function and capsid maturation by ribozyme targeting and electron cryomicroscopy. *Proc. Natl. Acad. Sci. U. S. A*, 102(20), 7103-7108.

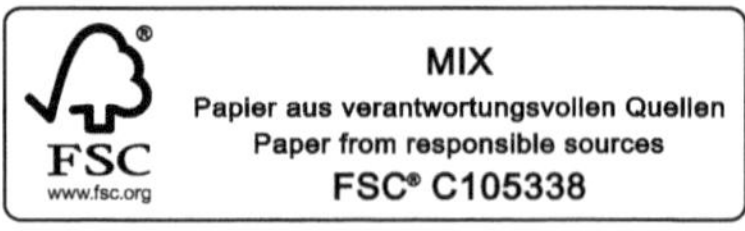

Printed by Books on Demand GmbH, Norderstedt / Germany